THE
MAGIC
OF
SEX

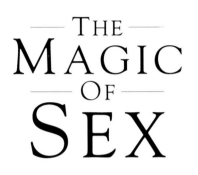

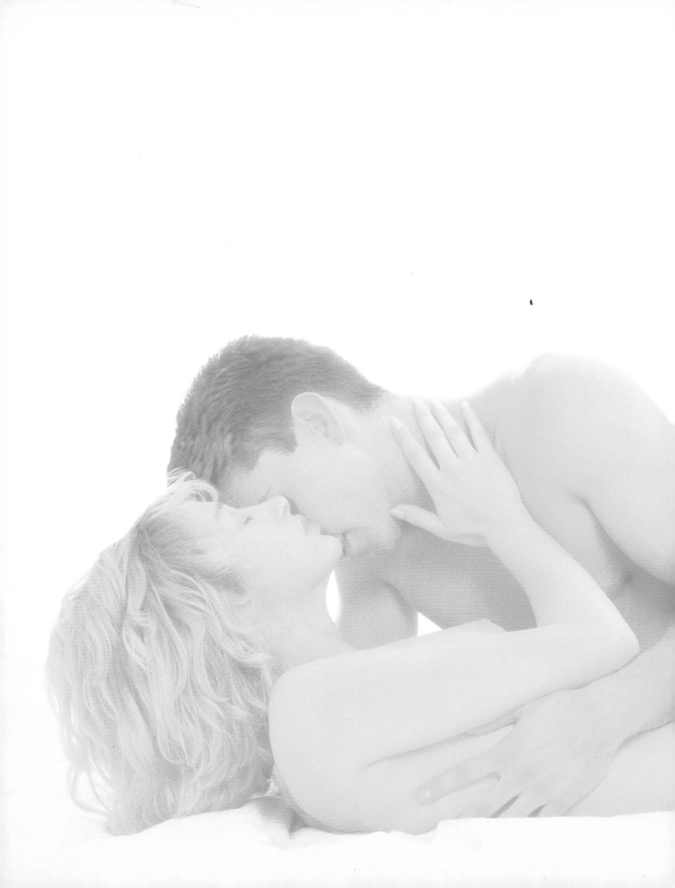

THE — MAGIC — OF SEX

MIRIAM STOPPARD, M.D.

DK PUBLISHING, INC
www.dk.com

"For TCOTB"

DK

A DK PUBLISHING BOOK

www.dk.com

Created and Produced by
CARROLL & BROWN LIMITED
12 Colas Mews
London NW6 4LH

First American Edition, 1992

17 19 20 18

DK Publishing Inc., 375 Hudson Street
New York, NY 10014

Library of Congress Cataloging
in Publication Data
Stoppard, Miriam.
    The magic of sex/Miriam Stoppard.
        p.   cm.
    Includes index.
    ISBN 1–56458–045–8
    1. Sex instruction. I. Title.
HQ31.S896   1992
613.9'6—dc20   91–29292
                            CIP

Reproduced by Colourscan, Singapore
Printed in Hong Kong

FOREWORD

For sex to be magic it needs the participation of both partners, and both partners should play as equal a part as possible. Yet, as you will see, the sexual partnership is one where the key players have differing abilities, propensities, responses, and reactions. A man's experience of sex is quite different from a woman's, and a woman's wants and needs may not mirror those of a man.

Therefore, to make this book as useful as possible, I have looked at every subject from both the man's and the woman's points of view, and the design carries this through. Under the male and female symbols, you will find information that is for or about men or women, as appropriate. Here I might write about the responses a man or woman has, what sexual activities he or she particularly likes, how he or she may want to be stimulated, what sensations he or she may feel, and so on.

And because so much of sex is about the bodily changes that can't be shown in any other way, I have used special color diagrams to chart sexual response, the varieties of sexual experience, and particular case histories that chronicle common sexual problems. Using normal sexual response as a benchmark, I've shown how experiences outside of it compare — whether better, as with multiple or prolonged orgasm, or worse, as with premature ejaculation.

Problems with sex tend to be unique to a couple, so in order to make the most of your sex life, you and your partner should assess your own predilections and activities, using the series of questionnaires I've devised, and then take the appropriate action as recommended within.

The magic of sex is there to be experienced by every couple. As you browse through the pages of this book, I am certain that what you discover about yourself and your partner will enable you to conjure the magic up, or show you where it has gone.

CONTENTS

INTRODUCTION:
SEX CAN BE MAGICAL 8

MAN AND WOMAN: THE SEXUAL PARTNERSHIP

ATTRACTION, AROUSAL, AND MAKING ADVANCES

THE MANY VARIETIES OF FOREPLAY

THE EXPERIENCE OF MAKING LOVE

LOVING SEX THROUGHOUT LIFE

HAVING IT ALL IN YOUR SEX LIFE

SUCCESS WITH YOUR SEXUAL PROBLEMS

REPRODUCTION, CONTRACEPTION, AND SEXUALLY TRANSMITTED DISEASE

SEX CAN BE MAGICAL

It expresses something that nothing else can, and it is the primary way of showing love. It is as important as, or even more important than, any other aspect of our relationships, be they long or short term. Beyond recreation and procreation, sex is the time, place, means, and language of knowing someone else on a level different from all others.

Primary, too, is the importance men and women hold for each other — something many of us have lost sight of. Loving partners give the kind of support that no one else can; very often they are the only ports in a storm. They provide emotional back-up, they help us to feel worthwhile, useful, and desirable. A loving partner makes one feel like a mature, well-rounded person with every chance of happiness. And in this context, sex is of paramount importance, because only a loving partner can give it. It is, therefore, the responsibility of every partner to do it well, because in the end, it is the one way of ensuring that a beloved companion will stay, and a loving relationship, with all its rewards, will last.

But having a good sex life is not about sexual athletics, physical agility, or just learning a series of sexual skills. This is why many sex manuals simply don't work; they emphasize the technical skills related to sexuality instead of the people involved. Experimenting with different techniques and positions does not guarantee that you will become a more sophisticated lover. The best lovers find out what their partners' preferences are; they do not necessarily indulge in sexual athletics. Good lovers are aware of the importance of closeness and caring; they desire to give love, and to give pleasure.

KNOWING ABOUT SEX IS IMPORTANT

Many people are very successful in their voyages of sexual discovery with the help of sympathetic loving partners who are open about their sexual needs, who are prepared to initiate and experiment, and who have the strength of character to know what they want, to verbalize it, and to get it by give and take. Those lucky people probably do not need a book of any kind.

But a book of this kind can be very important and useful to us all. It may rescue you if you are one of a couple where error inhibits trial, if your partner is not as understanding as he or she should be, if one of you has a temperament that is over-anxious rather than calm, and over-emotional rather than rational.
Or, you may have been conditioned to believe that certain sexual practices are right or wrong, better or worse, allowable or not allowable, and you will find another point of view enlightening.

Reading this book may also lead to discovery. Finding out information about sex may reward you with awareness rather than ignorance, with consciousness rather than obliviousness, with predilection rather than distaste. All of these discoveries are worthwhile. They are worthwhile because good sex is very nice and very enjoyable. In a way, it is a gift. It is a tragic loss if some of us are unaware of the gift and do not know how to use it.

Most of us have been brought up to think that intercourse is the ultimate intimate sexual act. I think that we are beginning to accept this less and less; most of us now see intercourse as but one option among many intimate choices.

Most of us are also coming to believe that the best sex can only be attained in a truly loving relationship, and that such a relationship is one that is nurtured, pursued, and lasts the test of time. It is a relationship in which two partners are interdependent rather than independent. We have been so preoccupied with the physical side of sex and "doing it" that we have forgotten the considerable joys of what was known as "marital" sex, which is all about giving — giving love and oneself totally to another person over a long period of time. This kind of love is not static; it grows and changes and develops in both partners. It encourages candor, sympathy, feedback about one's own and one's partner's behavior. To the surprise of many, this increases desire and eroticism rather than diminishing it.

THE REAL MAGIC OF SEX

My book reflects this modern attitude — that the most fulfilling sex is found in stable, long-term relationships, and in that respect, it is a very old-fashioned book. It is simply unrealistic to expect satisfying sex with a large number of people during short sexual encounters. It is only possible during a long period of loving with one person. As long as sexual experiences are good they can improve vastly with repetition; there can be great joy in the sameness.

So that sexual experiences can remain good, or become even more pleasurable, I have included much practical information to help you. I have discussed the male and female sexual anatomy and physiology, talked about the predilections that men and women have, looked at the variety of foreplay and the many ways of making love, and have given frank tips on how to enjoy sex more. But, in essence, this book is about getting back to partners loving each other; it is an attempt to straighten things out.

Man And Woman: The Sexual Partnership

THE TWO SEXES

Both my scientific research and personal observations have convinced me that men and women are more anatomically and physically similar than are the males and females of most other species. Any two men or two women that you see are likely to differ more in stature, size and shape than does the average couple. What is particularly distinctive about men and women are their reproductive organs, and the developmental changes, apparent in their mature shapes, that are caused by the actions of their sex hormones.

BOY INTO MAN

The changes that mark a boy's physical development into a mature man, one who is capable of reproducing himself, begin in the preteen and early teen years and are completed when he is between 14 and 18. These pubertal changes — when boys become taller and more muscular, with wider shoulders, more developed genital organs, and with hair appearing on their genitals, underarms, faces, chests, arms, and legs — are caused by the action of hormones, particularly the male hormone, testosterone. The adult male, in addition to the characteristics below, has experienced his voice "breaking," due to the larynx enlarging and the vocal cords becoming longer and thicker, causing the pitch of the voice to drop, along with an increase in sweat and sebaceous gland activity.

After testicular activity is established at puberty, it normally continues for the rest of life with only slight impairment in later years. There is a slight reduction in sperm and androgen production in old age, and this is associated with some degenerative changes in the testes, but there is no abrupt testicular decline comparable to the female menopause.

The "average" man is 5 feet 9 inches (173 cms) tall, weighs 162 lbs (74 kilos); his chest, waist, and hip measurements are 39, 32, and 37 inches (98, 80, 93 cms).

GIRL INTO WOMAN

In the latter part of adolescence, usually well after menstruation has begun, a girl's body begins to take on its female shape. (Prior to puberty, girls and boys, except for their external genitalia, are very similar.) The changes that occur are directly related to the secretion of the female hormones estrogen and progesterone. A girl becomes taller, her hips and thighs get fleshier, and she is more rounded and curvier. Her breasts begin to swell and hair starts to grow under her arms and between her legs. Her internal and external genital organs grow and develop, and the vaginal wall starts to thicken. Vaginal secretions may appear.

A woman's ultimate shape, be it curvaceous or boyish, is dependent on two things: first, the amount of hormones she produces, and second, the sensitivity of her body in reacting to these hormones.

Around the age of 45, ovarian function gradually wanes, and levels of estrogen and progesterone decline, resulting in bodily changes including cessation of menstruation and the loss of fertility, the thinning of the vaginal walls, and, very often, bone changes that result in a loss of height.

The "average" mature woman is 5 feet 3½ inches (158 cms) tall, weighs 135 lbs (61 kilos), with bust, waist, and hip measurements of 36, 30, and 38 inches (90, 75, 95 cms).

A MAN'S BODY

SKELETON

Beginning at about age 2, boys grow about 2 inches per year until age 13 or 14, when the sex organs begin to develop. Adolescence brings with it a sudden rapid gain in height, strength, and accompanying stature. The growth spurt that accompanies puberty may last for a few years, and during that time most boys gain about 3 ½ inches yearly. At the end of this period of growth, the bones have grown harder, more brittle, and change in proportion, different parts of the body grow at different rates. Once the shoulders start to broaden, the hips look narrower by comparison, and this appearance characterizes the adult male.

BODY HAIR

Early in puberty, pubic hair appears at the base of the penis, and after a while, it starts growing on the scrotum as well. It may also grow around the anal area. Pubic hair normally grows in an upside-down triangle on the lower part of the belly, though it may reach the navel, and may grow outward toward the thighs. About one or two years later, hair will appear in the armpits and on upper lips. Pubic hair is longer, coarser, and curlier than hair that has been present on the body since birth. It may be a lighter or darker color than that on the head. With age, it may turn gray.

In addition to curly pubic hair, hair appears on the arms, thighs, and lower legs. Hair may appear also on the chest, shoulders and back, and back of the hands. Facial hair becomes thicker and darker as a man matures. The beard and mustache may be the same color as the hair on the head, or different.

The amount of body hair is determined by a man's racial or ethnic background and family history. Caucasian men generally have more body hair than men of other groups, and "hairiness" runs in families.

A WOMAN'S BODY

SKELETON

Starting around age 2, a girl grows at an average rate of a couple of inches a year. About the time she reaches the age of 10, she experiences a growth spurt and begins to grow at a faster rate, perhaps gaining 4 inches or more in a single year, but then slows down again until she reaches her final height about one to three years after the onset of menstruation. While her bones are growing longer, not all grow at the same rate. Arm, leg, and foot bones grow at a faster rate than, say, spinal bones, and the pelvic bones take on a characteristically wide shape.

A woman has a wider pelvis than a man, in order to accommodate a growing baby, and her thighbones are set wider apart. This means that most women have knock-knees to some degree. The thighs have to slant quite steeply inward for the knees to come near the center of gravity.

BODY HAIR

Sexual body hair usually appears around the eleventh or twelfth year, just after the breasts have begun to grow. Pubic hair is longer, coarser, darker in color, and curlier than one's normal childhood hair, which has been present on the body since birth. Pubic hair first appears on the vulva and gradually spreads over the mons and vaginal lips, forming an upside-down triangle. In some women, pubic hair grows up toward the navel and out onto the thighs.

Women differ in the amount of pubic hair that grows — some have a lot, for others it is sparse. It can be any color and does not have to match that on the head. As a women ages, her pubic hair may go gray.

Almost two years after the appearance of pubic hair, more hair appears in the armpits.

MAN AND WOMAN

Genitals
The male genitalia, the penis and the scrotum, are located externally and are easily identified symbols of male sexuality. The female genitalia, however are mostly internal, hidden by pubic hair and less easily recognized.

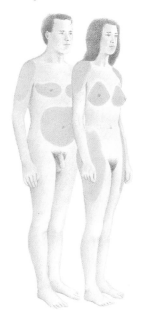

Fat distribution
A woman's body is 20-25% fat, which is mostly distributed on the breasts, hips, and thighs. A man's body is about 10-20% fat, distributed on the upper body and abdomen.

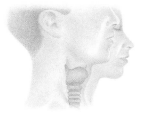

Voice
At puberty, the male vocal cords elongate and thicken; the voice "breaks" and lowers several tones. The thyroid cartilage enlarges and appears as the Adam's apple.

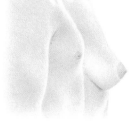

Breasts
These secondary sex organs are the same in males and females until puberty, at which time the male breast remains immature and the female breast develops— the areola swells, the nipple enlarges, the production of glands and fat increases.

Body hair

Early in puberty, males and females start to grow body hair. Girls grow pubic hair in an inverted triangle on their genitals, and hair appears in their armpits as well. Boys grow hair over much more of their bodies. The penis, scrotum, and anus are usually the first areas to grow hair, followed by the armpits and the upper lip. In addition to the pubic region, hair also appears on the arms, thighs, and lower legs.

HEALTH AND LIFE EXPECTANCY

The average life expectancy for both men and women has increased in the last few decades due to a decline in disease-related mortality. A woman's life expectancy is, on the average, about 80 years, and a man's is about 72 years.

STRENGTH AND STAMINA

Generally, men have a heavier bone structure than women and more muscle bulk, which accounts for up to 40-45% of body weight. However, despite their larger lungs and hearts, men do not necessarily have greater stamina than women.

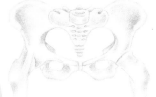

Male pelvis

Female pelvis

Pelvis size

The female pelvis is relatively wide and shallow to accommodate a baby during pregnancy. The larger and heavier male pelvis must support a greater body weight.

A MAN'S BODY

MUSCLES

The thighs, calves, shoulders, and upper arms begin to grow broader during adolescence, and strength increases, too. A grown man's muscles are 40 times their size at birth. The main determinant of body strength is body size, and muscle itself accounts for 40 percent of total body weight.

THE GENITALS

The testes grow very slowly until the age of 10 or 11, after which there is a marked acceleration in growth rate and growth of the external genital organs. In the fully grown male, the testicles are usually about $1^1/_2$ inches (3.8 cms) long, between 16 and 27 milliliters in volume, and are duskily colored. One testicle, usually the left one, hangs lower than the other. This is to keep the testicles from crushing each other when a man walks. In most men they are the same size, but in a few, one may be larger than the other.

Changes to the penis begin at a later stage than for the testicles. During a growth spurt, the penis gets larger — both longer and wider — and the glans, or head of the penis, becomes more developed. A grown man's penis is usually between 3 to 4 inches (7.5 to 10 cms) long when flaccid.

Under certain conditions, such as coming in contact with cold water or being out in cold weather, or feeling afraid or tired, a man's penis can shrivel somewhat temporarily. Old age, however, can cause it to become a bit smaller in size permanently.

A WOMAN'S BODY

MUSCLES AND FAT

Fat begins to be deposited on the breasts, hips, thighs, and buttocks when a girl is about 9 to 10. Later on, when a girl is about 15 to 17, more fat appears on the same areas . While her hips become rounded, the waist becomes curved and well-defined. Some women develop stretch marks, purplish or white lines on their skin, at this time. This happens when the skin is stretched too much during this period of rapid growth.

THE GENITALS

A man's genitals lie on the surface of his body where they easily can be seen and handled. A woman's genitals, however, are relatively inaccessible, more numerous, and fairly complex in design. Just as in other areas of anatomy, the genitals of women are individual; they come in a variety of shapes, sizes, colors, and textures. The genitals are covered in more detail on page 24.

BREASTS

The breasts are a symbol of feminine identity, forming part of the body image. Designed to nourish an infant, they are far more highly regarded by society as a source of eroticism, a symbol of femininity, a determinant of fashion, and a measure of beauty.

The breasts, or mammary glands, are modified sweat glands. Each woman's breasts are unique in their size, shape, and appearance, and this variation not only occurs between women but in the same woman at different times of her life, i.e. during the menstrual cycle, pregnancy, and lactation. Very frequently one breast is larger than the other.

In the center of the breast is a ring of skin called the areola; in its midpoint sits the nipple. The nipple and areola can range in color from a light pink to a brownish black.

SEXUAL ANATOMY

There is no doubt in my mind that an awareness of and familiarity with sexual anatomy can make you a better lover. Knowing where your partner's most sensitive areas are, how they are likely to respond to stimulation, and what happens when they do means that you will be able to give him or her maximum pleasure. And, if you realize that your partner is an individual who certainly will respond to particular caresses, perhaps in a particular way, your lovemaking will become much more effective.

—— YOUR GENITALS ARE UNIQUE ——

Men find it somewhat easier to understand their own sexual anatomy because their sexual organs hang outside and are clearly and constantly visible. But women and men both have less familiarity with female anatomy, and this is because so many of the important parts lie within a woman's body.

Just as in other areas of anatomy, the genitals of men and women are individual; they come in a variety of shapes and sizes. Normal variation means that there are a few women with exceptionally large or small vaginas, just as there are occasional men with exceptionally large or small penises. Women rarely express dissatisfaction with the size and shape of their external genitals — maybe because comparison with others is difficult, so ignorance is bliss. However, the vast majority of men are dissatisfied with the quality of their sex organs, and many feel that a small or average penis is a drawback to their sexual value.

Fortunately, there are many women who couldn't care less or who hardly notice the size of their partners' penises. Indeed, some women are physically uncomfortable with big penises; smaller penises are easier to handle when it comes to oral sex, for instance. Furthermore, many of a woman's sensations from intercourse come from the clitoris and from the nerve endings that are mainly in the first couple of inches of the vagina, so size really is irrelevant. It is a man's skill and patience as a lover, not the size of his penis, that is responsible for giving his partner sexual satisfaction.

On the other hand, many women are dissatisfied with their breasts and it may be that some of the dissatisfaction that both sexes have regarding their visible anatomy is the result of foreshortened viewing — both penises and breasts normally are viewed from the top down. What really matters, though, is taking pride and delight in your own individuality, and not worrying about what your genitals look like compared to others', and knowing that everything functions normally.

THE MALE SEX ORGANS

A combination of organs goes to make up male sexual anatomy; some of them are visible and some hidden. The visible parts include the penis and scrotum, in which the testes and epididymides lie. Those parts hidden from view include the prostate gland, the seminal vesicles, and the vas deferens.

THE STRUCTURE OF THE PENIS

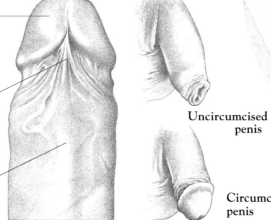

The glans (head)
Has a very thin skin that contains numerous nerve endings, and is extremely sensitive to touch.

The frenulum
The small piece of skin on the underside of the penis where the glans meets the shaft can be a man's most sensitive spot.

The shaft
The thicker the penis, the more likely it is to stimulate a woman's labia minora, and thus bring about orgasm.

Uncircumcised penis

Circumcised penis

The penis
Despite its mythical status, there is only one "universal truth," and that is each penis is individual. Erect penises, though they follow the same biological pattern, vary naturally in size, shape, color, length, angle of erection, and in the shape of the head. These variations have little effect on sexual sensation or performance.

The appearance of flaccid penises also may vary markedly, particularly depending on whether the foreskin is present.

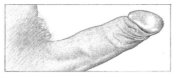

Blunt shape

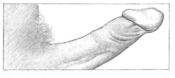

Bottle shape

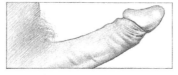

Prow shape

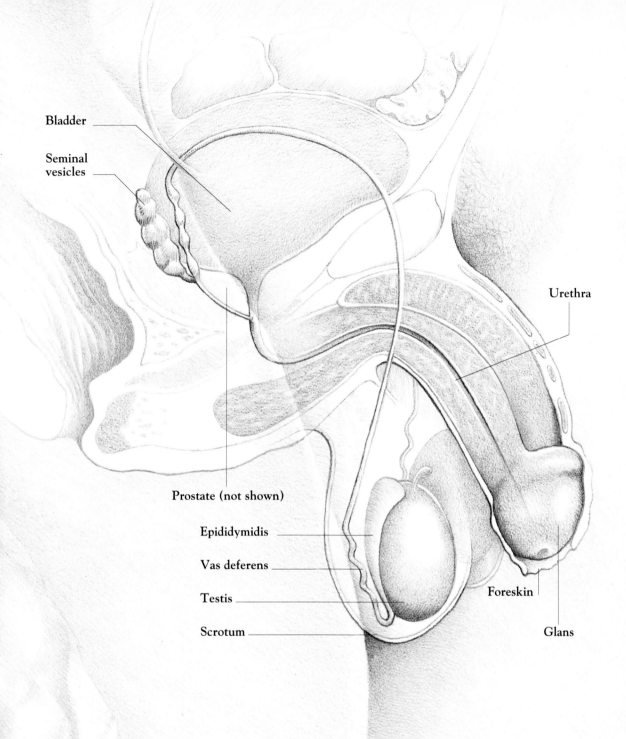

Bladder

Seminal
vesicles

Urethra

Prostate (not shown)

Epididymidis

Vas deferens

Testis

Scrotum

Foreskin

Glans

A MAN'S SEX ORGANS

THE PENIS

No organ has had so many myths perpetrated about it as the penis. It has been praised, blamed, and misrepresented in art, literature, and legend since time immemorial. Our own culture, too, has been influenced by, and responsible for, gross misconceptions of the performance and function of the penis. These phallic fallacies have not only been compounded in our art, but have become fixed in our culture, thereby influencing our attitudes and behavior.

The penis has two functions — the passage of urine and the deposition of semen in the vagina. Both of these are physiological and indisputable. But it is the role of the penis as the organ responsible for orgasm in both men and women that has achieved mythical status.

Penises vary in size, the average being 3¾ inches (9.5 cms) in the flaccid state. They are composed of erectile tissue arranged in three cylindrical columns; two on the back, the corpora cavernosa, and a single one underneath, the corpus spongiosum, which expands at the end of the penis to form the glans. Through the center of the corpus spongiosum runs the urethra, a narrow tube that carries semen (and urine) out of the body through an opening at the tip of the glans. When a man has an erection, and for a few minutes after, the urethra becomes compressed so that he cannot urinate, although semen can get through.

All of these structures are covered by muscles. The corpora cavernosa and spongiosum are filled with a rich network of blood vessels and blood spaces; the latter remain empty when the penis is flaccid but have the potential to fill and expand with blood during erection, hence the description cavernosa.

The expanded glans is demarcated from the main shaft of the penis by an indentation that runs around the head of the penis, the coronary sulcus, and the skin on the shaft of the penis forms a fold, the prepuce (foreskin), which extends from the coronary sulcus to cover the glans. On its lower side, the fold is tethered to the inner surface of the glans by the frenulum. This tiny band of very sensitive skin is, for many men, their most sensitive part and if stimulated, may quickly arouse them.

At birth, the foreskin is attached to the glans, but, starting in infancy, it gradually separates. The foreskin may be removed in a surgical procedure known as circumcision, performed for religious or hygenic reasons. There is no truth in the notion that an uncircumcised man can control ejaculation more effectively than a circumcised man. This myth is founded on the widespread misconception that the glans of the circumcised penis is more sensitive to touch or masturbation than the glans covered most of the time by a foreskin. During coitus, the foreskin retracts, exposing the glans exactly as with a circumcised glans.

The skin of the penis is thin, stretchy, completely devoid of fat, and loosely attached to the underlying tissues. The penis is richly supplied with sensory nerves and also with nerves from the autonomic nervous system that lodge in the pelvis.

CHANGES TO PENIS SIZE

Normally, the penis increases in size — an additional 2¾ to 3¼ inches (7 to 8 cms) — and stiffness when a man is sexually aroused. Erection may take place in a few seconds, and is due to a very great increase in blood flow into the penis. The blood spaces in the corpora cavernosa and spongiosum fill with blood, which is prevented from draining away into the veins by swollen arteries that compress them, and thus the erection is maintained until after ejaculation takes place.

It is widely accepted that the larger the penis the more effective a man is as a sexual partner. This delusion, for it is a delusion, that penile size is related to sexual potency, is based on yet another phallic fallacy — that when a larger penis becomes erect it achieves a bigger size than does erection of a smaller penis. But this is not the case. In Masters and Johnson's laboratory, men whose penises measured 3 to 3½ inches (7.5 to 9 cms) in length in the flaccid state increased by an average of 3 to 3¼ inches (7.5 to 8 cms) at full erection. This full erection essentially doubled the smaller organs in length over flaccid size standards. In contrast, in the men whose organs were significantly larger in the flaccid state — 4 to 4¾ inches (10 to 11.5 cms) — penile length increased by an average of only 2¾ to 3 inches (7 to 7.5 cms) in the fully erect state.

THE SCROTUM

The scrotum is the pouch of skin, situated below the root of the penis, that houses the testes. It is divided by a fibrous sheet, and this division can be seen on the surface of the scrotum as a ridge, the scrotal raphe. The scrotal skin is dark and thin and contains numerous sebaceous glands and sparse hairs. Under the skin is a smooth muscle, the dartos muscle. This muscle contracts in response to cold or exercise, and its contraction makes the scrotum smaller and its skin wrinkled.

THE TESTES

The testes are smooth oval structures compressed from side to side like broad beans. The left testis may be situated at a slightly lower level than the right testis. Each testis is inside a sac and has four coverings corresponding to the various layers of the abdominal wall; these are carried down into the scrotal sac when the testis migrates from inside the abdomen just before birth. Small muscles called cremasters control the height of the testes. The position

of the testes may change according to a man's level of sexual arousal, his emotions, and the temperature of the scrotum, among other things. If sperm are to develop normally, they must be produced at a temperature two or three degrees lower than the rest of the body. That is why the testes are "outside" the body.

The testis has two functions: to produce sperm and to produce male hormones or androgens, primarily testosterone. The epididymis is a comma-shaped structure that is stuck to the rear surface of the testis, its tail being continuous with the ductus deferens. This fine tube carries sperm developed in the testis to the epididymis where it is stored. The epididymis is, in effect, an extensively coiled duct, which if straightened would be 5 to 7 yards long.

The vas deferens then transports sperm via the spermatic cord into the pelvis, where it joins the back of the bladder with the seminal vesicle. Each duct then continues downward and, joined by the duct of the seminal vesicle, forms the ejaculatory duct, which runs on through the substance of the prostate and enters the male urethra inside the prostate gland. Each seminal vesicle contains 2-3 ml of sticky fluid in which the sperm are supported and nourished, and which forms the ejaculate.

THE PROSTATE

The prostate is a fibrous, muscular, and glandular organ having the shape of a chestnut. It produces secretions that form part of the seminal fluid during ejaculation. It is contained in a fibrous capsule and is situated just below the neck of the bladder. The male urethra passes right through the center of the prostate. This means that if the prostate gland enlarges, the urethral outlet may be narrowed, leading to difficulty in passing urine, dribbling, and poor stream, a not uncommon condition in men over the age of 55. Beyond the prostate are the pair of Cowper's glands that also add lubricant to the seminal fluid prior to ejaculation.

THE FEMALE SEX ORGANS

The female sex organs are highly complex, and to most people they are more of a mystery than the male's, since they are less accessible to the eye because of their largely interior positioning.

   The external organs, the opening to the vagina and its surroundings, are collectively known as the vulva or pudendum. This highly sensitive and erotic area is bounded by the mons pubis at the front, the perineum at the back, and the labia majora and minora at the sides.

THE STRUCTURE OF THE VULVA

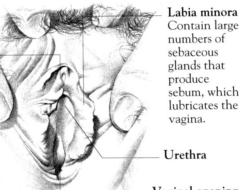

Clitoris
Contains receptive nerve endings to make it the most erotically sensitive part.

Labia majora
Covered by pubic hair, they contain sebaceous and epocrine glands.

Labia minora
Contain large numbers of sebaceous glands that produce sebum, which lubricates the vagina.

Urethra

Vaginal opening

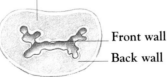

Cross section of the vagina
Shows an H-shaped cavity that has great expansive capacity.

Front wall

Back wall

The vulva
Like most other parts of the human body, the vulva is highly individual and varies from woman to woman in appearance and in its areas of greater or lesser sensitivity. The external appearance differs most obviously in the size of the labia majora and minora.

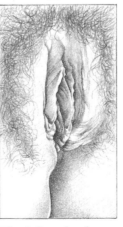

Thick-lipped vulva

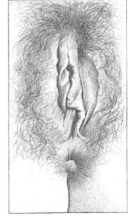

Thin-lipped vulva

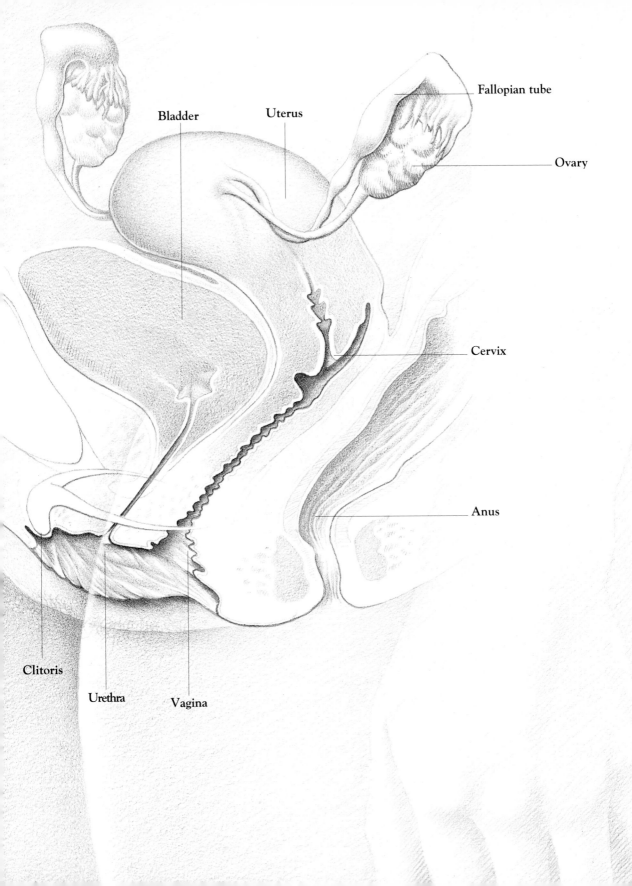

Bladder

Uterus

Fallopian tube

Ovary

Cervix

Anus

Clitoris

Urethra

Vagina

A WOMAN'S SEX ORGANS

THE VULVA

A woman's external and visible genitalia are known as the vulva or pudendum. It is a very erotic area, highly sensitive to touch, which also serves to protect the vaginal and urethral openings. The fatty tissue and skin at the front of the vulva is the mons pubis, sometimes called the mound of Venus; it covers where the pelvic bones join at the front (the symphysis pubis), and acts as a cushion during intercourse. In the mature female, the mons pubis is covered by a triangle of hair.

The most superficial structures of the vulva, the labia majora, extend forward from the anus and fuse at the front in the mons pubis. These "lips" are twofold and normally lie together and conceal the other external genital organs. They are composed of fibrous and fatty tissue, and carry hair follicles and sebaceous and apocrine glands. The latter give rise to a particular form of odorous sweat, which is a sexual chemical attractant and stimulant for most men. They are regarded by some as the female equivalents of the male scrotum, the left one being slightly larger than the right.

The labia minora are folds of skin that lie between the labia majora. Unlike the labia majora, the labia minora contain neither fat nor hair follicles, but they have large numbers of sebaceous glands that produce sebum that lubricates the skin and, in combination with the secretions from the vagina and sweat glands, forms a waterproof protective covering against urine, bacteria, and menstrual blood.

There are wide variations in the size and shape of these lips and, like the labia majora, one is generally larger than the other. They may be hidden by the labia majora or project forward. During sexual excitement they become engorged, change color, and increase in thickness — sometimes as much as two to three times normal size.

THE CLITORIS

The clitoris (key, in Greek) is the most sensitive organ of the vulva and is the female equivalent of the penis, having the same component parts in miniature. In anatomical and physiological terms, the clitoris is a unique organ. No organ which acts solely as a receptor and transmitter of sensual stimuli, purely to initiate or elevate levels of sexual tension, can be found in the human male.

The body of the clitoris is ¾ to 1¼ inches (2 to 3 cms) long and is acutely bent back on itself. The top of clitoris is covered by a sensitive membrane that contains many receptive nerve endings. During coitus, the clitoris doubles in size and becomes erect — in exactly the same way as the penis. The length of the whole clitoris, including the shaft and glans, varies greatly depending on stimulation by hormones during puberty.

THE HYMEN

In childhood, a thin membrane, the hymen (named after the Greek god of marriage), guards the opening to the vagina. It is normally perforated and so allows the escape of menstrual blood. Its thickness and stiffness vary from woman to woman; in rare cases it is so strong and resistant that intercourse is difficult and the hymen must be cut under local anesthetic. Normally, however, it is torn during childhood activities such as gymnastics, cycling, or horseback riding, or occasionally by the use of tampons. Even if intact, it is rarely so painful during first penetration as literature would have us believe.

THE VAGINA

Many myths, not to mention jokes, surround vaginal size. The vagina is a potential, rather than an actual space. It is a fibro-muscular tube measuring about 3¼ inches (8 cms) in length, but its size is variable, and so flexible that any normal vagina can accommodate any size of penis with ease. If penetration occurs early, before expansion in length and diameter is complete, a woman may experience initial difficulty in accommodating an erect penis, particularly a large one. But vaginal expansion continues rapidly so that the penis, regardless of size, is accommodated with the first few thrusts.

As excitement climbs, the vagina normally over-extends in length and over-extends in circumference. This elliptical vaginal expansion accounts for some loss of stimulation for the penis, and reduces vaginal sensation for the woman, giving many women the sensation that the fully erect penis, regardless of size, is "lost in the vagina."

——— INSIDE THE VAGINA ———

The projection of the cervix allows the space of the vaginal vault to be divided into front, back, and lateral fornices. The cervix enters the vault through the upper part of the front vaginal wall and as a result, the front wall is shorter than the rear wall and the rear fornice is much deeper than the front one. This arrangement favors the passage of sperm into the cervix during intercourse because when a woman lies on her back, the opening of the cervix is not only directly exposed to semen, but is bathed by the pool of ejaculate which forms in the posterior fornix in which it rests. During intercourse, it is this posterior fornix which takes the brunt of penile thrusting and so protects the cervix from injury.

The lining of the vagina is thick and is thrown into prominent folds called rugae, some of which run longitudinally and some horizontally. The lining cells of the vagina contain glycogen, a kind of starch. The fermentation action of bacteria, which normally live in the vagina, on the glycogen produces lactic acid that renders the fluid in the vagina on the acid

side of normal. This acid environment is necessary to maintain the health of the vagina and deters bacterial growth. Any interference with the delicate ecological balance, for instance vaginal douches, can cause irritation, inflammation, discharge, and allergic reactions.

The lining of the vagina does not contain glands, even though the vagina lubricates itself with a kind of sweat when sexually aroused. Under normal circumstances, cells that are routinely shed from the lining of the vagina, plus mucus secreted from the cervix, plus vaginal sweating, form the normal vaginal discharge, which is colorless and odorless. The vagina contains a muscle coat which runs mainly longitudinally, and it is richly supplied with blood vessels. Its action opens or closes the vaginal space. Inside the top of the vagina, directly behind the pubic bone, is said to be an area of erectile tissue, which when stimulated produces a different type of orgasm. This area, known as the G spot, is discussed in more detail on page 36.

THE GREATER VESTIBULAR GLANDS ——— AND URETHRA ———

The greater vestibular glands (Bartholin's glands) lie behind and slightly to the side of the vagina. The ducts of these glands open into the angle between the labia minora and the ring of the hymen and carry lubricating mucus to the vaginal opening and the vulva's inner parts.

The urethra is intimately embedded within the substance of the lower half of the front vaginal wall, so that bruising of this wall can result in inflammation of the urethra and an ascending infection of the bladder (cystitis). The middle third of the rear wall of the vagina is closely related to the rectum, and the muscles which form the pelvic floor, the levatores, blend with the middle part of the sides of the vagina, forming the most crucial support of the vaginal structure.

THE ACT OF INTERCOURSE

Pleasurable sexual intercourse depends upon both partners passing through stages that result in the necessary erection for penetration with sufficient lubrication to receive it, the stimulation of penis, vagina, and clitoris to achieve orgasm, orgasm itself, and the gradual winding down of the body's responses and return to normal.

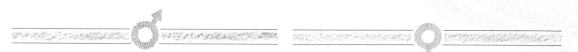

THE MAN'S EXPERIENCE

THE WOMAN'S EXPERIENCE

Arousal
Responding to physical and mental stimuli, the erectile tissues fill with blood and the penis becomes firm and erect.

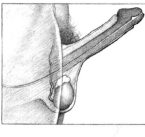

Arousal
Under the influence of foreplay and other stimuli, lubrication occurs, the clitoris lengthens, and the vagina enlarges.

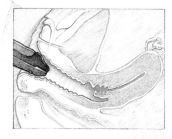

Plateau phase
Once inside the vagina, the man begins thrusting movements; his penis is at its maximum size and his testes have elevated.

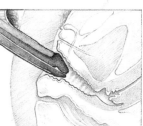

Plateau phase
If penetrated, the muscles of the walls of the vagina contract and grip the penis. The uterus rises and the clitoris retracts under its hood.

Orgasm
Muscular contractions propel semen out of the penis during ejaculation and result in intensely pleasurable bodily sensations.

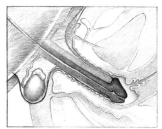

Orgasm
The vaginal walls contract strongly and rhythmically several times, and intense sensual feelings spread throughout the body.

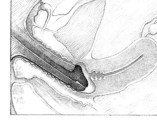

Resolution
The penis loses its erection and the testes descend to their normal position. It will take a man some time to become erect again.

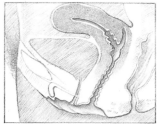

Resolution
Gradually, clitoral and labial swelling diminish, and the vulva and vagina return to their normal size and color.

The "Missionary" Position

In the most common position for sexual intercourse, the woman lies on her back and the man enters her from above.

Pressure caused by being sandwiched between the pelvic bones of both partners stimulates the clitoral area

The entire length of the penis enters the vagina

The vagina expands to accommodate the penis; the back wall receives the most stimulation

SEXUAL RESPONSE

If we are attuned to our bodies, we know that sexual response has identifiable stages — desire, arousal, climax, and resolution, and that these are accompanied by bodily changes. What is less well known is that although these stages occur in men and women in the same order, and in much the same way,   there are vital differences. For

A WOMAN'S RESPONSE TO SEX

Exciting a woman brings about changes in many different parts the body. As a woman becomes sexually aroused, her breathing becomes more rapid, and her heart beats more quickly. Her lips become pink, the pupils of her eyes dilate, and her nipples become erect. As excitement climbs, her skin becomes pink and flushed, it begins to sweat, and her breasts swell as they become engorged with blood.

—— THE VAGINA BECOMES MOIST ——

But a woman's first response to sexual stimulation, which is usually tactile, is vaginal lubrication, which can appear within 10 to 30 seconds of excitement; individual droplets of mucuslike material appear at intervals throughout the folds of the vaginal walls. (This ongoing lubrication is actually a form of sweating). While the clitoris is the primary focus of a woman's sexual response, its reaction is slower, and nowhere near the speed of penile erection.

As sexual excitement increases, the droplets fuse together to form a smooth, glistening, lubricating coat over the entire barrel of the vagina, making penetration by a penis extremely easy. This lubricating mucus can appear in the most copious amounts, despite the absence of glands in the vaginal walls, and it is thought to originate from an enormously increased blood supply, which is almost simultaneous with the onset of sexual excitement. No other source for the mucus has been discovered. The response is almost certainly not hormonal,

as it occurs in women who have had a complete hysterectomy.

—— THE CLITORIS RESPONDS ——

The speed of response by the clitoris depends on whether it is stimulated directly or indirectly. The most rapid response depends on direct stimulation of the clitoral body or the mons area. Indirect stimulation, including manipulation of other erogenous zones such as the breast or vagina, without direct clitoral contact, has a definite but slower response.

The only form of direct stimulation is touch — by the fingers, mouth, or penis, and most women require some in addition to penetration to achieve orgasm. Because of its position, the clitoris is not stimulated directly during intercourse, so movements of the penis on its own are often insufficient to excite the clitoris to orgasm. However, indirect stimulation of the clitoris does develop with penile thrusting, the body being pulled downward and then the hood being released, and along with breast and vaginal stimulation, should occur in every coital position.

—— THE VAGINA CHANGES ——

As sexual excitement increases, the shape of the vagina changes in readiness for penetration. The inner two-thirds of the vaginal barrel lengthens and distends; sometimes expansive movements occur. In highly excited women, this distention is quite marked. (Such expan-

women the changes are usually initiated by different stimuli and take a longer time to occur, but they last longer and can be repeated more quickly. The changes are reversible if either party is distracted.

Desire, the recognition that our feelings and sensations are taking a sexual turn, begins in the brain, which then sends messages to the body that result in a variety of changes indicating arousal. Arousal, if prolonged sufficiently, leads to climax, and with orgasm, muscular tension is released and the flow of blood to the pelvis is reversed.

---

sion is involuntary, and the walls relax in an irregular and flexible manner.) The cervix and uterus are pulled backward and upward into the pelvis, further expanding the upper end of the vagina.

At the same time, the color of the vaginal walls alters. Under normal conditions, the vagina is a deep pink, but this color slowly changes to a darker purplish hue, as the blood supply to the vagina increases.

In the preorgasmic state, the vagina is so distended that all the folds of the wall are stretched and flattened, and the lining becomes thin. In the plateau phase, the outer one-third of the vagina swells with blood, and this distention may be so great that the lower part of the vagina is reduced by at least a third. Increased blood supply also results in enlarged labia minora and majora, which become separated, elevated, and turned out.

ORGASM OCCURS

It has never been possible to study the orgasmic changes in the clitoris due to its retraction beneath the hood formed by the labia minora. The changes in the vagina, however, are much easier to study. The outer one-third contracts regularly during orgasm, there normally being three to five, up to a maximum of ten to 15 contractions at 0.8 second intervals. After the first three to six contractions, the space between them lengthens. Each contraction is intensely pleasurable, and these fantastic sensations fall away as the contractions lessen.

The duration of orgasmic contractions, their degree, and the space between them varies from woman to woman and from one orgasm to another. Occasionally, with the highest tension levels, orgasm may start with one profound contraction lasting two to four seconds before the muscle spasms develop into the regular contractions lasting less than a second.

During orgasm, the uterine muscle contracts, and the fornices expand, forming a tent to receive the sperm.

THE BODY RETURNS TO NORMAL

After orgasm it takes some time for the vagina to return to its normal appearance. As long as ten to 15 minutes may elapse before the basic coloration returns to the vagina, and for the folds to reappear.

The clitoris returns to its normal overhanging position within five to ten seconds after orgasmic contractions have ceased, and the discoloration of the labia minora disappears just as quickly: in fact, these two things mirror the loss of erection after male orgasm. Detumescence of the clitoral glans is a relatively slow process and may last five to ten minutes; in some women, it may take as long as 30 minutes. If orgasm isn't reached, swelling of the clitoris may last for several hours after sexual activity.

A MAN'S RESPONSE TO SEX

When a man becomes excited, his reactions, just like a woman's, are not confined solely to his sex organs. Excitation starts in the brain, when a man becomes aroused by something either real or imagined. A man is aroused by predominantly visual stimuli; he is "turned on" by clothing and makeup, as well as the sight of naked or seminaked female bodies. A man readily becomes conditioned by his experiences; objects or circumstances associated with sex may elicit arousal, too. In this way, without any physical contact, male arousal occurs frequently and rapidly.

THE PENIS BECOMES ERECT

Messages from the brain travel down the spinal cord to the genitals and shut off the outflow of blood from the penis, and this brings about an erection. A man's normally limp, downward-hanging organ becomes a rigid, upward-pointing, dusky colored, throbbing one with prominent veins.

By carefully controlling the variation and intensity of stimulative techniques, erection can be maintained for extended periods; it can be partially lost and rapidly regained many times during a long period of stimulation.

Erection can be easily interrupted by nonsexual stimuli, even though sexual stimulation is continued. A sudden loud noise, a change in lighting or temperature, or any form of mental distraction may result in partial, or even complete, loss of erection.

INTERNAL AND EXTERNAL BODILY CHANGES OCCUR

In addition to causing the penis to become erect, the increased blood supply leads also to reddening and mottling of the skin in about a quarter of all men. This "sex flush" starts in the lower abdomen and spreads over the skin of the chest, neck and face. It may appear on the shoulders, forearms, and thighs, and, when fully developed, may even resemble measles. Its appearance is always evidence of high levels of sexual excitement. After ejaculation, the sex flush disappears very rapidly — initially from the shoulders and extremities, and then from the chest, and finally from the neck and face.

A man's breast, like a woman's breast, is responsive to sexual stimulation. Though the pattern is inconsistent, nipple swelling and erection, which may develop without direct contact and may last for an hour after ejaculation, occurs frequently. Many women are not aware that a man's nipples, and even his chest, can become erogenous zones if they are given enough stimulation.

A man's heart rate increases with sexual excitement, and his respiratory rate and blood pressure also rise. His scrotum thickens and his testes will be drawn closer to his body. Many men sweat involuntarily immediately after ejaculation, but this is not proportional to the amount of physical exertion during sexual intercourse. Sweating is usually confined to the soles of the feet and the palms of the hands but may appear on the trunk, head, face, and neck.

A FEELING OF INEVITABILITY IS EXPERIENCED

Immediately prior to orgasm, there is a sense of ejaculatory inevitability for an instant. Many men describe the onset of this sensation as "feeling the ejaculation coming." From the onset of this sensation there is a brief interval, two to three seconds at most, during which a man feels the ejaculation coming but no longer can prevent, delay, or in any way control the process. This subjective experience of inevitability develops as seminal fluid is collecting in the prostatic urethra, just before the actual emission of seminal fluid begins. While a woman's orgasm can be interrupted by extraneous stimuli, once initiated, a man's orgasm cannot be delayed until emission has been completed. Despite the intensity of extraneous distractions, the male must keep going until completion.

Just prior to ejaculation, the glans penis may change color; its mottled, reddish-purple color may deepen. (This is reminiscent of the preorgasmic discoloration of the labia minora in a woman.) A drop of fluid may form at the urethral opening of the penis prior to ejaculation. This is not seminal fluid but secretions from Cowper's glands (see p.21). The size of the testes increases marginally and they also become elevated. At this point, it is increasingly difficult for the penis to return to its resting state without ejaculation.

Muscle contractions occur late during sexual excitement and may be involuntary but possibly voluntary depending on body position. Spasms of a man's hands and feet can occur — rarely if the man is "on top" — but more commonly when he is supine.

─────── ORGASM OCCURS ───────

Regularly recurring contractions of the urethra and the deep muscles of the penis result inevitably in ejaculation and the exquisitely pleasant sensations of orgasm. The entire length of the penile urethra contracts rhythmically and forces seminal fluid from the full length of the penis under pressure, often for some distance. During ejaculation, contractions of the rectal sphincter occur simultaneously with the expulsive contractions of the urethra.

The penis contracts similarly to the vagina during orgasm: the contractions start at intervals of 0.8 seconds and, after three or four major expulsive efforts, they are rapidly reduced in frequency and in expulsive force. Minor contractions of the penile urethra may continue for several seconds in an irregular manner, projecting a minimal amount of seminal fluid under little, if any, force.

If a man has been abstinent for several days he generally ejaculates a larger volume of seminal fluid than when he is more sexually active. A larger volume is often more pleasurable than a lower volume, and this may account for a man's greater pleasure after a significant period of continence than after repeated orgasms. This pattern is the opposite of that reported by women who, as a rule, enjoy the second or third orgasm most.

Orgasm and ejaculation are two separate processes and may, or may not, occur at the same time. One can occur without the other. Orgasm involves the sudden pleasurable sensations and release of tension, which usually occurs in the genital area and elsewhere in the body; ejaculation involves the discharge of seminal fluid from the penis. A man may ejaculate as the result of sexual stimulation but not experience the sensation of orgasm. Less frequently, a man may have an orgasm but not ejaculate. Most men who experience multiple orgasms ejaculate only once.

─────── THE PENIS DETUMESCES ───────

Normally, the penis becomes flaccid following intercourse and a man will not get another erection for some time. If a man removes his penis from his partner's vagina immediately following ejaculation, full detumescence is accomplished much more rapidly than if his penis remains there. Just maintaining close physical proximity to his partner may prolong the second stage. Walking about, conversing about extraneous subjects, or other diversions can cause the penis to lose its erection with relative rapidity; urination will always increase the rate of penile detumescence since a man cannot urinate with a fully erect penis.

Once the penis returns to its normal size, the man will relax and very often feels sleepy.

ORGASM

Orgasm, the climax of sensation, is a uniquely human experience. For men, orgasm depends almost entirely on the stimulation of the penis, either by hand or mouth, as well as the vaginal walls, and is usually, though not always, accompanied by ejaculation of seminal fluid. For women, clitoral stimulation and movement of the penis within the vagina, prolonged through skill and experience, produce these intense feelings, though they can reach orgasm in other ways, too — by manual or oral stimulation of the clitoris, vagina, or G spot, for instance. About one woman in ten experiences the emission of fluid from the urethra with orgasm. It is thought that this fluid comes from the Skene's glands, which run alongside the urethra, since it is not urine or vaginal mucus.

Orgasms vary: mood, level of energy or fatigue, amount and type of loveplay, the level of mutual trust, and what is happening in either partner's life all have their effects on the sensation. And not every sexual experience can, or should, end in orgasm; there are times when orgasms are a natural outcome of sexual activities and others where lovers will have orgasms only if they really work at them.

A MAN'S ORGASM

— WHAT HAPPENS TO THE BODY —

As the engorged reproductive glands spurt out their contents into the part of the urethra that runs through the prostate, expanding it as they do so, exquisitely pleasant sensations are produced. A series of four or five contractions, at the rate of one every 0.8 seconds, follows as the man ejaculates stored semen.

Some men tend to have extremely powerful physical reactions during their orgasms, moaning and groaning, contorting their faces and bodies, and sometimes even scaring their partners by their cataclysmic reactions. Other men may have very tranquil, quiet orgasms leaving their partners wondering whether they have come at all. Most men probably experience a range of intensities between these two extreme reactions.

A WOMAN'S ORGASM

— WHAT HAPPENS TO THE BODY —

The duration of orgasmic contractions, their degree and the space between them, varies from woman to woman, and from one orgasm to another. Some women experience a high peak of pleasure that fades away rapidly; others feel it as a more widespread, warm, internal sensation, and still others arrive at a peak, which subsides gradually into a series of pleasurable plateaus.

In response to orgasm, a woman may arch her body, tense her muscles, and her face may be pulled into a grimace. She may scream, cry out, or bite her lips, or, her partner may just see a quickening of excitement, feel some involuntary hip movements, muscle contractions in the genital area, and a general release of tension as the orgasm subsides.

A MAN'S ORGASM

ARE THERE DIFFERENT TYPES?

We're just beginning to discover that like women, men have a variety of orgasms with the added differences that different patterns of ejaculation can provide. There is no right way for a man to ejaculate or to have an orgasm.

Often the main source of pleasure is a powerful ejaculation. On the other hand, the sensations of orgasm may be felt for a long time with the ejaculation experience almost as an anti-climax, yet on other occasions a man may experience a number of continued orgasmic sensations long after he has ejaculated, or a man may experience a pattern similar to the multiple orgasms of women — a series of fairly closely spaced mini orgasms with ejaculation occurring at the last.

IS MORE THAN ONE POSSIBLE?

After a major orgasm most men experience a refractory period during which further sexual stimulation does not lead to an erection. Many males below the age of 30, however, have the ability to ejaculate frequently with only short resting periods. While men are resistant to sexual stimuli immediately after ejaculation, with practice and learned control, many men can extend their sexual cycles and enjoy several mini-orgasms before a final climax.

After orgasm a man's emotional reactions most often reflect his relationship with his partner. Satisfaction, contentment, and happiness result from a loving relationship; sadness, depression, and a drained feeling can follow where intimacy and understanding are lacking, as in one-night stands. Most men, too, feel mentally drained after orgasm with the common result that sleep readily ensues.

A WOMAN'S ORGASM

ARE THERE DIFFERENT TYPES?

Masters and Johnson told us categorically that the origin of the female orgasm is in the clitoris and that there is not a second kind of orgasm that originates in the vagina. Research into the personal experience of many women does, however, suggest that at the very least there is a type of orgasm that starts in the clitoris and spreads down into the vagina, resulting in a more powerful climax than when the orgasm involves the clitoris alone. This kind of orgasm is said to result from stimulation of the G spot (see p.36) and is reputed to be deep, powerful, prolonged, and accompanied by contractions of the vagina, uterus, and pelvic organs. Women state that it is truly transporting and brings them in closer union with their partners than any other.

IS MORE THAN ONE POSSIBLE?

A major difference between the sexes is that many more women are capable of experiencing more than one orgasm during a single sexual act. By holding back from the brink or preventing themselves from ever reaching orgasm, men should be able to prolong coitus and give more than one orgasm to their partners. Instead of moving to the resolution stage, those women able to have multiple orgasms remain at the plateau phase in a highly aroused state, and from there they can be stimulated to orgasm quickly and repeatedly. However, just because a woman is capable of having multiple orgasms does not mean they will occur every time she has intercourse, or that she wants them to.

After orgasm, women are less prone to the slightly depressed feelings that men often have, and most welcome further loving attentions. A very few women experience a drifting into a mild form of unconsciousness, poetically known as the "little death," after orgasm.

CHARTING SEXUAL RESPONSE

THE MAN'S EXPERIENCE   After only a few minutes of stimulation, excitement increases quickly until the man reaches the plateau phase, where he can remain for any length of time according to his desires. Most men have to remain here for several minutes, sometimes 30, but on average about 15, until their partners catch up and penetration becomes mutually desirable. Once inside, a man's sexual pleasure increases markedly, especially as thrusting movements bring him steplike to the point of no return and an intensely pleasurable moment with orgasm and ejaculation. After this, excitement drops steeply, the penis becomes flaccid, and he enters the refractory period, a variable time during which an erection is no longer possible.

ORGASM

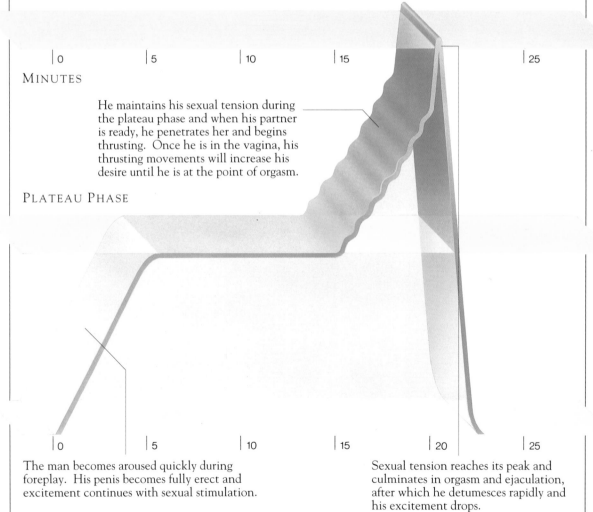

MINUTES

0   5   10   15   25

He maintains his sexual tension during the plateau phase and when his partner is ready, he penetrates her and begins thrusting. Once he is in the vagina, his thrusting movements will increase his desire until he is at the point of orgasm.

PLATEAU PHASE

0   5   10   15   20   25

The man becomes aroused quickly during foreplay. His penis becomes fully erect and excitement continues with sexual stimulation.

Sexual tension reaches its peak and culminates in orgasm and ejaculation, after which he detumesces rapidly and his excitement drops.

THE WOMAN'S EXPERIENCE Sexual tension in the initial stage increases slowly, frequently taking 20 or 25 minutes but, on average, 15 minutes. The more varied and stimulating the foreplay, the more rapidly a woman passes through this initial arousal phase. Her pleasure then rises in a parallel and stepwise fashion with the thrusting of the penis within her vagina. If direct stimulation of the clitoris is maintained throughout this period, a woman can proceed quickly to the point of orgasm. After orgasm there is a slow and gradual return to normality, often extending up to half an hour. During this resolution phase, the breasts return to their normal size and the swelling of the labia diminishes.

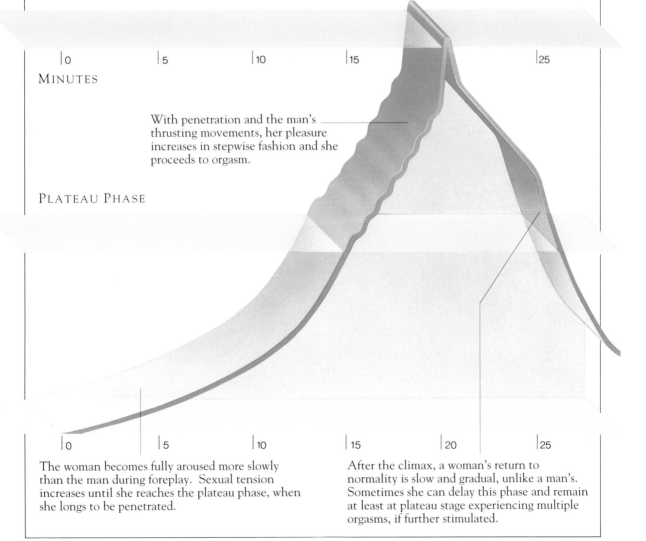

ORGASM

MINUTES

| 0 | 5 | 10 | 15 | | 25 |

With penetration and the man's thrusting movements, her pleasure increases in stepwise fashion and she proceeds to orgasm.

PLATEAU PHASE

| 0 | 5 | 10 | 15 | 20 | 25 |

The woman becomes fully aroused more slowly than the man during foreplay. Sexual tension increases until she reaches the plateau phase, when she longs to be penetrated.

After the climax, a woman's return to normality is slow and gradual, unlike a man's. Sometimes she can delay this phase and remain at least at plateau stage experiencing multiple orgasms, if further stimulated.

THE G SPOT

In Germany in the 1940s, an obstetrician and gynecologist called Ernst Grafenburg, researching new methods of birth control, claimed to have discovered a new, internal zone of erogenous feeling in the women he was studying. This sparked a controversy, which has become more heated in recent years, concerning the existence of these male and female G (Grafenburg) spots.

Stimulating the G spot
A face-to-face sitting position such as this enables the penis to stimulate the front wall of the vagina, where the female G spot is located.

There seems to be little doubt that there is a hidden area, at least in some men and women, which when stimulated produces intense excitement and orgasm; in women this has become known as the G spot, and in men is identified as the prostate gland. While it is physiologically undeniable that men have a prostate gland, pathologists have failed to find the G spot (which feels like a small bean when stimulated), when performing postmortems on females. Some experts believe that it is possible that the G spot exists only in some women; others believe simply that the front wall of the vagina is very sensitive and when stimulated can produce an orgasm in some women; others dismiss the whole idea as complete nonsense and claim that the entire controversy causes unnecessary feelings of inadequacy and anxiety among both men and women.

Self-discovery is really the only way to find out if the G spot can produce intense pleasure for you or whether, as for some people, it is a complete waste of time.

THE MALE G SPOT

The male G spot has been identified as the prostate gland, which, like the female G spot, is situated around the urethra at the neck of the bladder. The prostate gland has an organic function helping to produce the fluid which carries sperm into the vagina during intercourse. Many men discover that stimulation of the prostate before or during intercourse can result in an extremely intense orgasm, during which they ejaculate in a gentle stream rather than in spurts.

It is very difficult for a man to find his own G spot, or prostate gland, since the only way for him to feel an internal gland is through the anus. The best position for discovering the gland yourself is to lie on your back with your knees bent and your feet flat on the floor, or with your knees drawn up to your chest. Insert your thumb into the anus and press against the front wall. Your prostate should feel like a firm mass about the size of a walnut, and when stimulated, should produce feelings of intense sexual excitement.

THE FEMALE G SPOT

The G spot appears to be a small cluster of nerve endings, glands, ducts, and blood vessels sited around a woman's urethra, or urinary tract. This area cannot normally be felt when unaroused, only becoming distinguishable as a specific area during deep vaginal stimulation. When this happens it swells, sometimes very rapidly, and a small mass with distinct edges stands out from the vaginal wall. As it appears to have no organic function other than helping a woman achieve a high degree of sexual fulfillment, and, at orgasm, can appear to "ejaculate" a clear liquid similar in composition to that created by the prostate, some experts believe that the G spot is a rudimentary form of the male prostate gland.

The easiest way for a woman to find her G spot is to sit or squat, as lying down positions the relevant spot further away. It is best to begin your explorations while sitting on the toilet since first stimulating your G spot can feel like a desire to urinate. Once the bladder is empty, you will feel comfortable going on knowing that the sensation is caused by the G spot, and not by having a full bladder.

THE MALE G SPOT

STIMULATING THE MALE G SPOT

The anus is delicate, unused to having things inserted in it, and not a naturally lubricating organ. In order not to cause damage, ensure that fingernails are short and that fingers are well lubricated with KY jelly or a similar substance.

If you want your partner to stimulate you, lay down on your back and have her gently insert a finger into your anus. Allow yourself enough time to become accustomed to having her finger there, then have her feel up the front rectal wall until she finds your prostate and massages it firmly. Then she can stroke the gland in a downward direction. This can be tiring to both partners but is made a little easier for the man if he pulls his knees back toward his chest. Without her even touching your penis you will probably become erect and have an orgasm.

This maneuver is not as "messy" as a woman may perhaps think, since unless you are constipated, there are no stools in your lower rectum. Your partner must, however, wash her fingers at once and must not touch inside her vagina, or you could transfer bacteria. Some women feel better using a disposable plastic glove, especially since it protects against transmitting the AIDS virus.

Some women like to fellate their partner while massaging his prostate, and you might suggest this to your partner as well.

THE FEMALE G SPOT

STIMULATING THE FEMALE G SPOT

Using your fingers, apply firm upward pressure on the front of the internal vaginal wall, perhaps pressing down simultaneously with the other hand on the outside of the abdomen. As it becomes stimulated, the spot should begin to swell and will feel like a lump between the fingers inside and outside of the vagina. Pleasurable contractions may sweep through the uterus and you may experience a deep orgasm, which will feel totally different from a clitoral orgasm.

At this point you also may ejaculate a small amount of clear fluid from the urethra, which, despite appearances, is not urine.

It may be more effective if your partner stimulates you since he can reach the spot more easily. Lie down on a bed with two pillows underneath your hips, with your legs slightly apart and your bottom a little in the air. Your partner can lean close against you, gently insert two fingers, palm down, and stroke the front vaginal wall.

Sexual positions that produce G spot stimulation are the woman-on-top and the rear-entry positions. In the latter, the penis is rubbing directly on the front wall of the vagina in which the G spot is located. When a woman is on top, she can control the depth and direction of her partner's penis, and can move forward or side-to-side to guide it to the place that feels best.

A man can help by moving his own body and pressing the base of his penis to make sure that the head makes full contact with the G spot. The result can be a series of intense orgasms for both partners.

Attraction, Arousal, And Making Advances

YOUR APPEARANCE

While there may be many ways of enjoying sex, most people will enjoy sex more if they are sure of themselves — not simply sure of what they are doing, but sure of their attractiveness and desirability.

Attractiveness or sex appeal is very hard to define, but sexuality has more to do with your attitude toward yourself, your partner, and your lifestyle than anything else, and certainly more to do with these than with obvious physical attributes. We have all met rather plain, unassuming people who have enormous charm and charisma, which is difficult to pin down but often has to do with having a positive attitude toward life, a ready smile, a subtle sense of humor, and being enthusiastic. Other people are attractive because of their eccentricity and uniqueness — a way of speaking or expressing themselves, mannerisms, surprising candor, or individualistic presentation.

Such qualities are more important than your actual appearance, and while it is worth spending some time on how you look, you should maintain a sense of balance by not becoming obsessive about your physical appearance. Too many men and women feel dissatisfied, not because they have gross or obvious abnormalities, but simply because they compare themselves to an exaggerated image of what is good looking. Responding to your partner, being flexible about his or her preferences, and being willing to share pleasure are the qualities that ultimately make a person attractive.

Although excessive attention to appearance isn't necessary, some relationships can founder if either partner neglects his or her appearance and hygiene. The best possible reason for being careful about your appearance is for your own self-esteem, but you should also do so for your partner's sake; otherwise he or she could interpret neglect as a sign of not caring. This does not imply that one has to spend hours on preparation, but an unclean and smelly body, dowdy ill-kempt clothes, an unshaven face, curlers in the hair, and a bad-tempered face all imprint themselves on the memory and become difficult to erase at times of intimacy. A sloppy appearance invites comparison with the time when you first met, and the inevitable thought arises that love is on the wane.

— LOOKING AT YOURSELF POSITIVELY —

Many people find it worthwhile to take a good, hard look at themselves as a way of getting in touch with and appreciating their bodies. Most of us are far too hard on ourselves and it will boost your ego quite a bit if you, for a moment, concentrate on your good points rather than emphasizing your bad points.

Doing the following should help to lessen self-consciousness and make you more comfortable with yourself and with your body as a source of sexual pleasure. It is best to do these "exercises" in private, when you have plenty of time and feel as relaxed as possible.

MAN'S SELF-APPRAISAL

1 Undress in front of a full-length mirror and examine your naked body carefully, from head to toe. Imagine you are seeing yourself for the first time. Look at yourself from every angle.

2 Stand, kneel, bend, and move around. Sit with your legs apart and then together. Look over your shoulder to see the curve of your back and the set of your buttocks.

3 Focus attention on your best points; everybody has some. They might be the breadth of your chest, the flatness of your stomach, your height, or the fullness of your hair.

4 Then pay attention to the features that you dislike and try to see them in a more positive way. For instance, while you may think yourself shorter than ideal, you may be trim and perfectly proportioned.

5 Now study your genitals. Feel your testes; one, usually the left, will hang slightly below the other. Your flaccid penis will probably be between 2 and 4 inches (5 to 10 cms) long and, when you touch it, you will find the most sensitive area is the head and, in particular, the ridge on the underside.

6 Finish by taking a warm bath. Soap your hands and explore your body with them, noticing the different sensations you experience with changes in touch and pressure. Explore your penis and testicles again, too, if you like, but try to become aware of sensations throughout your whole body.

WOMAN'S SELF-APPRAISAL

1 Stand naked in front of a full-length mirror and examine your body carefully from head to toe as though you were seeing yourself for the first time. Use another mirror to see yourself from the side or back.

2 Move around. Kneel, bend, and sit with your legs apart and then together.

3 Concentrate on your best points — we all have some. The shapeliness of your legs, the length of your neck, high cheekbones, or dainty feet may be yours.

4 Reconsider the features that you dislike and try to see them in a more positive way. For instance, while you may think yourself fatter than ideal, you may have a Rubenesque physique that is attractive to men.

5 Using a hand mirror and, in the best possible light, study your vagina. Identify your different parts. In order to see and touch the clitoris properly, you will need to pull back the hood of skin covering it. You can run your fingers along the inner and outer vaginal lips and back along the area between the anus and vagina to find the more sensitive areas. Separate the inner lips in order to explore the entrance to the vagina and inside.

6 When you have finished, take a warm bath. Soap your hands and explore your body, using them to notice the different sensations you experience in all your body areas by changes in touch and pressure.

ATTRACTING A PARTNER

Both our ability to love and our style of loving begin to develop from the moment we're born. Scientists believe that many of the associations we form in infancy help determine whom we choose as sexual partners or soul mates and that patterns which lay down tendencies for love relations are etched into our brains.

I can show you how this might be so by looking at how just one of the senses, smell, predetermines a particular choice. Each of us, even in our highly deodorized society, has a unique odor that is the sum of our glandular secretions — a "smell signature." Whether our smell signature is attractive to other people — because it reminds them happily of their mothers, for instance — or turns them off, because it reminds them of detested ex-spouses, say, depends on those people's own associations. Associations are linked to smell because the olfactory bulb involved with smell reception feeds into the part of our brain that is linked with emotion and affective memory.

In the same way, we can learn to like the smells of our loved ones. Studies have shown that lovers can pick each other out of a group solely by their unique aromatic signatures (and that is how babies first bond with their mothers). If we lose our ability to smell, we normally suffer a pronounced slump in sex drive.

THE CHOICE OF A PARTNER

Highly personal patterns like our individual smell associations make it extremely difficult to generalize about attraction. Men and women, in general, are attracted to the sexual characteristics that separate them — for example, women's larger breasts, men's broader shoulders. Cultural expectations, too, have a large role to play; a man to whom a French woman would be attracted is probably very different from a Chinese woman's ideal partner. Age, social class, personality, and what we want from a particular partner also very much determine whether or not we find a person attractive.

Many myths exist as to what men and women find attractive in each other. There is no proof, for example, that gentlemen prefer blondes; in fact, studies have shown that dark-haired men prefer brunettes, and fair-haired men like brunettes and blondes equally. And, while men think women like men with hairy chests and large penises, most women mention tenderness, affection, respect, sensuality, and kindness as a man's most attractive qualities. If pressed, women will generally admit to preferring dark-haired men of average build, with small buttocks and a tall, slim physique. A large penis is not important; in fact, penis size is rarely mentioned.

WHAT WOMEN LOOK FOR IN MEN

The choice of a partner still is determined very much by evolutionary patterns whereby women first looked for mates who could be relied upon. For that reason, physical appearance appears to be less important to women than personal qualities. Women like men's bodies for what they represent — protection, power, or comfort — not as sex objects.

Age is not so determining a factor in a woman's choice of a man. Unlike men, who usually look for younger women (subconsciously aware that older women may be incapable of childbearing), women can be attracted to men of all age groups; younger women may like older men, older women often seek younger men.

PERSONALITY   Confidence, assertiveness, independence, and dominance are generally found appealing, as are reliability and faithfulness, and qualities that suggest warmth, intimacy, and attentiveness. Men who try to get along with women and talk freely and openly about what interests them, and use a soothing voice, are more successful with women.

PROWESS   Men who are successful at work or sports, and have the visible proofs, are more likely to attract women.

PHYSICAL QUALITIES   A man who is fit and healthy, with a degree of leanness and a well-muscled body that is not scrawny, and who may have some surprising feminine characteristic such as long eyelashes, is considered more attractive than a stereotypical muscle man. Women prefer men taller than themselves.

PERSONAL CHARACTERISTICS   A body cleansed of the sweat of the day and free of body odor; a genital area whose scent is not too pungent; well-cared-for hands; well-washed feet and a clean pair of socks daily; clean hair; a face that is clean shaven or with a shapely beard and without a rash are what will attract.

WHAT MEN LOOK FOR IN WOMEN

Men generally place a higher premium on physical appearance than women do. In surveys, physical attractiveness is number one on the list. Women's bodies are often on display in advertising and magazines, and men have been conditioned to find certain attributes particularly stimulating. Legs, for example, are powerful attractants because they indicate the state of a woman's maturity; high-heeled shoes, stockings, and skintight pants emphasize their allure and reinforce their sexual imagery. A woman's more pronounced female buttocks, narrow waist, bare shoulders, and lips all act as sexual signals, but her breasts are her most obvious turn-on. Men, however, differ in what exactly they find attractive. Some men even describe themselves as leg, buttock, or breast men. By and large, men are attracted to women younger than themselves — perhaps a subconscious recognition of childbearing capacity.

PERSONALITY   Traditional traits such as warmth, sympathy, kindness, gentleness, and cheerfulness are often cited as desirable. Erotic ability is more highly rated than domesticity.

PHYSICAL QUALITIES   A degree of leanness with a curvaceous outline, rather than thinness, is desired over a more maternal figure. A narrow waist and long legs are universally admired, but breast size and shape are individual tastes (see above).

PERSONAL CHARACTERISTICS   A genital area that is not too pungent or whose natural smell is not masked by deodorants or other synthetic smells; shapely polished fingernails and well-cared for hands; not too much body hair (a woman's legs are smoother and more pleasant to touch if hair is removed); clean, soft hair; clean-smelling breath with no nicotine aroma — these are what attract men.

MAKING ADVANCES

Sending out messages requires directness and a certain degree of vulnerability. It nearly always requires self-esteem to take the knocks and rejections we might receive when we make an advance. We need to have a mixture of arrogance and humility to assume that someone would want to know us better, while remembering that many people might rather have nothing to do with us. We ask ourselves the questions: "Do I remember taking this risk before and was it comfortable or uncomfortable?" "Am I prepared to take this risk again?" An encouraging thought is that it is rare for someone you are interested in to be entirely indifferent to you.

WHERE AND HOW TO MEET

Many people think that there are only certain social situations where sex can be on the agenda. However, this is not true; any situation can lend itself to sexual advances. Of course, in some situations, advances need to be subtle and very low-key; in fact, difficult to pick up unless the other person is sexually aware and alert.

Only someone with a closed mind would limit his or her horizons to parties, dinners, and social occasions. Sexual interest can be revealed at any time. For instance, a working business meeting between two sexually interested people, when each may be thrilled by the other's professional performance, can be an exciting and intriguing prelude to more open sexual overtures. Here, the enjoyment of a common task can enhance sexual interest greatly. Indeed, sexual interest grows more often in the day-to-day working environment than almost anywhere else.

While women rate nightclubs and dances as the most likely way of meeting men with whom they would like a sexual relationship, reality is different. Most people meet potential sexual partners through friends, and like any other form of friendship, most happy sexual relationships are based on friendship and on working or studying together. You can get to know someone better at work than in a nightclub. Furthermore, when looking very glamorous and affected by drink, we don't necessarily give a realistic picture of ourselves, nor are we able to get an insight into a partner.

A less obvious advance could occur when you have lunch with or talk to someone over a period of time in a quiet spot. Glances are often exchanged and conversations may include messages with a double meaning, testing how interested the other person is. These interactions may just be in the form of play, but all of us do engage in them and establish brief "mini" bonds with many people.

SENDING OUT MESSAGES

The truth is we cannot *not* communicate. Even if we are not speaking, we are giving out signals through the body. People are perceived as being friendly or unfriendly without a word being spoken. Body gestures give messages about subconscious emotions and are, therefore, a very direct form of communication. You can use them to see what others are thinking. They often belie what we are saying; probably, nonverbal gestures are more accurate in many situations than words themselves. And, as we gain awareness of nonverbal behavior and an interest in interpreting the body language of others, we become aware of our own bodily gestures and this can result in more effective outward communication.

EYE CONTACT

By far the most common initial sexual advance is eye contact. Our eyes meet with interest, with approbation; a very brief fantasy may occur — "I'm sure I would like to have a relationship with you. I will never talk to you but I think we could be great together"— and we may think about this anonymous message later. These encounters may take place in the street, walking down the hall at work, on the stairs, in an elevator, or at a traffic light, and they happen often. We do this every day of our lives, even if we are very happy with a partner. We seem to keep practicing attraction by sending at least mini-messages to test our abilities.

Eye contact is one of the simplest and most direct ways of showing someone that you are sexually interested in him or her, and by making eye contact, you make it easier for that person to respond to you.

Always look at the person you are talking to, not over his or her shoulder or down at the floor. To show interest in another, hold your glance longer than you would do in an ordinary social situation, but don't overdo it. Most people find intermittent eye contact — about five seconds out of every 30 — most comfortable and will probably drop their gaze if you look at them directly for too long. A person expresses interest if he or she returns your gaze steadily.

VERBAL COMMUNICATION

Conversation, too, whether at a casual encounter, an intimate dinner, or during the course of work, can be a huge sexual turn-on. Glances are often exchanged and conversations may include messages with a double meaning that test the interest of the other person.

Expressing ideas, motivations, goals, and aims can bring two people closer together than many other activities. And where there are areas in common — similar interests, ambitions, and plans — this is very thrilling to both partners. The exchange of thoughts and ideas along these lines between a couple who are sexually aware of each other is, in my opinion, one of the most pleasant ways of initiating a sexual relationship, and it will also solidify the relationship once it has begun.

– FACIAL EXPRESSIONS AND GESTURES –

Another thing to remember in order to make certain you are sending out the right signals is keeping your facial expressions pleasant. Smiling is especially important because it is a direct way of telling someone that you find him or her attractive or pleasant to be with.

Using hand and head movements are also ways of encouraging people as they indicate interest in you. Make sure you stand the right distance away — physical proximity indicates attraction and is a cue for greater intimacy, while standing far away points to mistrust and aloofness.

Finally, learning to use touch to communicate can step up the pace of any relationship. To give a positive response in the early stages, touch your partner's arm while talking to him or her or, if you come up from behind, put a hand on his or her shoulder in greeting. Bear in mind that you should keep it subtle. You don't want to overstep the line between showing interest and being too pushy or pawing. Remember, too, that skin-to-skin contact — touching a bare forearm with your finger, for instance — is always much more intimate than skin-to-clothing contact.

When you want to increase the pace further, move on to more prolonged and frequent touching — holding hands, for instance, and from purely social gestures like brushing hands as you give something over to more overtly sexual ones, like lingering pressure on the palms.

JUDGING RESPONSES

By paying attention to body language (see pages 48-49) and other signals, you should be able to see if you are having a positive effect on the other person. Encouraging responses include raised eyebrows, wide-open eyes, and dilated pupils. A definite "come-on" signal is if you are looking into each other's eyes for longer and longer periods, and if you are standing close as you do so. You can test this by moving slightly closer and seeing whether the other person draws away (negative) or not (positive). Watch the gestures your partner makes; if he or she nods the head in enthusiastic agreement at what you are saying, or if he or she touches you to emphasize a point when talking to you, you are making progress!

RESPONDING TO AN ADVANCE

Responding to a message requires a lowering of defenses, and some risk-taking. Acknowledging that an invitation is being sent out to you is one of the riskiest steps. Most of us find ourselves thinking, "How well can I trust my senses, even my own ears?" "Have I interpreted the intonation of what is being said correctly; does that person really mean what he or she is saying?" "Why should that person be interested in me?" "Maybe it is just a joke, a tease; will I look like a fool if I take this seriously? But, and it is a big but, will I hate to miss the chance just in case it is serious and I would like to go further?" When an invitation is perceived, all of these thoughts can occur almost simultaneously to the person receiving the advance.

Once an encouraging message is sent, received, and acknowledged, each person is on his or her best behavior and projects the kind of person that they think would please the other. It is only later that partners begin to show their true colors and test how their relationship might work in everyday life with its stresses and strains.

SOME POINTERS FOR MEN

Social responsiveness is not the same as sexual encouragement. And invitations can be misunderstood. For instance, when you're invited to someone's apartment for the first time and told to make yourself comfortable, do you take off your jacket, loosen your tie, and lounge on the sofa? Do you let your anticipation show and then, when your date returns in jeans and an old shirt, do you feel foolish when she says, "What do you think you're doing, moving in? I've got to finish putting up my bookshelves. Why don't you get yourself a drink before letting yourself out; I don't want to mess up the kitchen."

Nor should you expect every encounter to lead to great romance or sex. If you get too serious or expect a woman to give more than she is prepared to, you will probably make her retreat. Many women prefer a softer approach to an overtly sexual come-on, and it is not a good idea to be familiar too soon. Express admiration and interest but stay away from endearments or physical caresses at first.

SOME POINTERS FOR WOMEN

Sexual relationships usually progress in small steps, with each of you giving, and in turn, responding to, signs of encouragement. Picking up and responding to the other's cues correctly will minimize the risk of your social responsiveness being interpreted as sexual encouragement.

It is important, too, to know exactly what you want out of a relationship. Many women are shy about admitting that they just want sex, not a long term loving relationship. Some women even will go so far as to generate feelings of love in order to have sex, and this, in the long term, will prove unsatisfactory for both you and your partner.

Nor should you expect every encounter to lead to great romance or sex. If you get too serious or expect a man to give more than he is prepared to, you will probably make him retreat. It is not a good idea to be familiar too soon. Express admiration and interest but stay away from endearments or physical caresses in the beginning.

BODY LANGUAGE

Body language is the process of communication through positioning — leaning toward someone; brief, accidental touches or bumping; leaning on each other; talking closely to someone so that your heads touch; showing skin, even perhaps just a wrist. The body goes through a dance, and as the body dances, it gives out messages. We are all very sensitive to these messages, particularly of "bonding" body language and nonbonding body language. At the same time, we discover or rediscover our feelings, which are subsequently reflected in our body movements and positions.

Our antennae don't take in single, unrelated gestures that are quite often misleading. What we take in is called a gesture cluster; that is, a set of related movements of the arms, feet, head, and inclination of the body, which together make up a meaningful message and significant interpretation. One gesture is akin to a single word in a language, and an isolated word is often meaningless. With gestures as with words, messages become clear only as a series is used.

The scenario below illustrates a newly introduced couple and the gestures that indicate their interest, or lack of it, in each other.

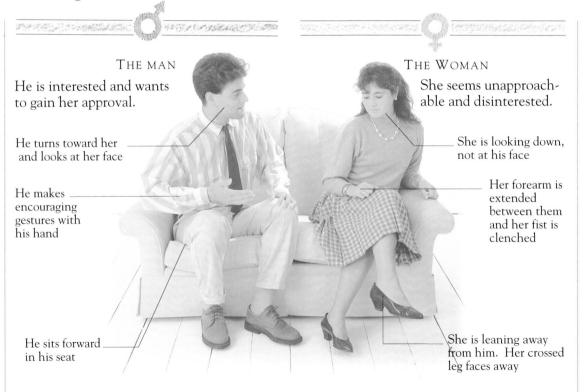

THE MAN

He is interested and wants to gain her approval.

He turns toward her and looks at her face

He makes encouraging gestures with his hand

He sits forward in his seat

THE WOMAN

She seems unapproachable and disinterested.

She is looking down, not at his face

Her forearm is extended between them and her fist is clenched

She is leaning away from him. Her crossed leg faces away

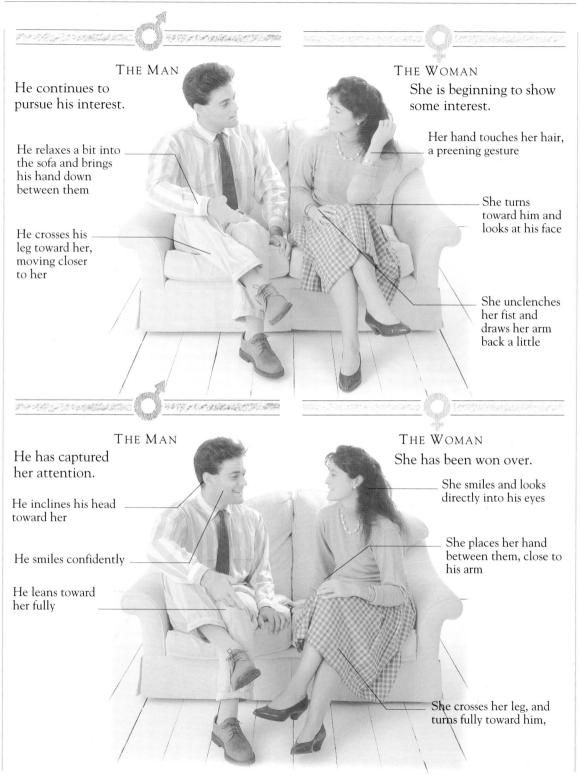

THE MAN

He continues to pursue his interest.

He relaxes a bit into the sofa and brings his hand down between them

He crosses his leg toward her, moving closer to her

THE WOMAN

She is beginning to show some interest.

Her hand touches her hair, a preening gesture

She turns toward him and looks at his face

She unclenches her fist and draws her arm back a little

THE MAN

He has captured her attention.

He inclines his head toward her

He smiles confidently

He leans toward her fully

THE WOMAN

She has been won over.

She smiles and looks directly into his eyes

She places her hand between them, close to his arm

She crosses her leg, and turns fully toward him,

AROUSAL

When we are attracted to or aroused by someone sexually, all our senses — but particularly sight, touch, and hearing — come into play. Our sense of smell, while important, plays a much smaller part than for other species. Traditionally, it has been the woman who attracts with visual displays of gestures and apparel, and the man who responds with sexual arousal, but changing patterns of sexual behavior has lead to a somewhat greater equality of role. For example, today both sexes wear clothes explicitly to attract the opposite sex — men with tight trousers and form-fitting tops, women with low-cut necklines and slim, short skirts.

In terms of the stimuli that excite them, men and women differ markedly. Men, generally, are stimulated by what they see. Women, on the other hand, are very different; as a general rule, they respond very little and very slowly to visual stimuli. Women are more interested in men in the context of their personalities.

———— WHAT TURNS US ON? ————

SIGHT This plays a greater role in arousing men than in women, but a woman may take advantage of this by making herself as visually attractive as possible, with makeup, flattering clothes, and by ensuring that her movements — such as when undressing — are pleasing to watch. The eyes are supposed to be the windows of the soul, so it is very common to see lovers gazing intently into each other's eyes, oblivious of everything else around them.

HEARING This contributes much, too, which is why music, played quietly and at the right moment, can be highly exciting for both men and women. We become excited when we hear our beloved approaching, his or her laugh, and particularly his or her voice. Some men and some women have very beautiful voices, and are aware of their seductive effects. A man may have a warm, velvety voice whose every modulation has the power to move a woman's heart. A good voice used well is a caress, and most lovers would wish to be caressed in this way for a long time. A telephone call may simulate an act of love and be as potent as any form of foreplay. The opposite pertains, too, of course, and some women's voices drive men crazy.

TOUCH Even small touches, even accidental touches, have an enormous effect on everyone. We all need touch very badly. We find it relaxing and reassuring, and it helps us to loosen our inhibitions. Sometimes the greatest intimacy and the most acute closeness can come from simply touching and holding. Most of us have had experiences where dancing has been highly erotic, involving the rhythmical contact of two bodies. Dancing can be pure foreplay — try dancing cheek to cheek, hand in hand, breasts against a man's chest, pelvis against pelvis, legs slightly apart, thighs brushing each other, sexual organs pressed together — all of which simulate sexual contact. The potent mixture of sight and sound created by movement, light, and music only adds to the effect.

TASTE This can play its part also — a good meal accompanied by good wine often puts a couple in a good mood and lowers their inhibitions so they are more inclined to make love. Talk over a meal, appreciating the softness of the light, and the ritual of eating, can be very seductive, and lovers feel that there is a metaphor between eating and deriving emotional nourishment from a partner's body.

SMELL Women like wearing perfume and men like smelling it, but it can have a much greater effect than a woman ever thinks — especially when her body is warm; the scent evaporates and body smells mingle with the perfume, and this can act as a powerful stimulant. It was Coco Chanel who first said that a woman should scent her body wherever she expected to be kissed, and with the array of scents available, both partners would delight in this. Women probably have the strongest preference for the unadulterated smell of a man's skin, which in itself is very exciting, but as a way of showing interest, most wouldn't mind if their partners used some aftershave.

WHAT MEN LIKE

BARE FLESH This is rated very highly by men. Exposed bodies and expressions of a "come hither" variety are extremely arousing.

MAKEUP Bright red lips are a sexual turn-on, as are other things connected with physical appearance, such as hair style and color.

SEXUALLY EXPLICIT MATERIAL Girlie magazines, soft-porn videos, and pin-up photos are very arousing and are used to feed fantasies and for masturbation. Most men, however, would not be much aroused by their own partner appearing in a girlie magazine; it is the fact that such a woman belongs to somebody else that is part of her attraction.

SEXY CLOTHING Black, lacy underwear and scanty nightclothes are particularly pleasing to most men. It is no mystery why models pose in garter belts and stockings.

WHAT WOMEN LIKE

PHYSICAL ATTRACTIVENESS While not necessarily at the top of the list, most women will confess to being attracted to certain aspects of their partners' bodies, though not normally their genitals.

POWER AND WEALTH Visible signs of dominance, which is expressed in today's world by being in possession of money and status, are turn-ons for the majority of women.

ROMANCE AND INTIMACY Other important aspects of setting that are arousing to most women are expressions and manifestations of a romantic interlude such as champagne, moonlight, and flowers.

EROTIC LITERATURE Many women will confess to enjoyment of erotic literature in the form of popular romantic novels. However, sexually explicit material has also been found to excite many women.

INITIATING SEX

While a few people believe that one-night stands are one of the most satisfactory forms of human relationships, the majority of us feel that, in addition to physical attraction, there has to be love, and love involves knowing someone. In fact, sex is the ultimate act of knowing. But in order to know someone, you have to show yourself. For the majority of people knowing is not easy; we feel vulnerable and open to the possibility of rejection, which can be extremely painful. But I don't believe that sex can ever be initiated without knowing one's partner and showing oneself. No relationship can thrive where these two basic ingredients are missing.

From the outset, we must tell the truth and nothing but the truth. Any other form of behavior is distancing and hypocritical; you must represent yourself honestly. In a loving relationship, even a white lie is an insult and extremely damaging. Honesty in itself is arousing; it can be a stimulant. Truth is probably the best aphrodisiac.

We're all vulnerable, both emotionally and romantically, so in a relationship that will involve love and sex you should declare your vulnerability. Don't forget that having sex is a decision as well as an impulse, and it does not mean that you have to lose control. It means letting your partner know that the basic reason for your being there is that you are looking for love; you are looking for someone to bond with. When we decide to have sex with someone we are being intimate with all they are; so declare all you are.

The myth of romanticized women and eroticized men distorts the natural interaction between the two sexes. The infinite range of human experiences through holding, touching, feeling, stimulating, trusting, and talking is involved in sexual interaction, and it is a distortion of the male and female personalities to say that love and sex are the sole prerogative of either gender.

SOME POINTERS FOR MEN

• Take some care over your appearance; never fall into bed unshaven and unwashed.
• Have something nice planned; almost all women appreciate a bouquet of flowers and candlelit dinners, for instance.
• Compliment your partner on her appearance, tell her she smells nice, hold her hand, give her affectionate kisses, and catch her eye and smile whenever you can.
• Be attentive whether you are out together alone or at a party; for example, don't ignore her for the television.
• Once you're in bed be attentive to her wishes and indulge in as much loving foreplay as you can.
• Try not to fall asleep immediately after you've climaxed; talk to her a while afterward and hold her in your arms.

SOME POINTERS FOR WOMEN

• In matters of love, go for it; don't dissemble and deceive. Nothing works as well as going all out after someone you want, and to keep on working at it once you are together. Going after someone means giving yourself.
• Take some care over your appearance; clean, well-cut, sweet-smelling, freely moving hair and an attractively made-up face can be very appealing.
• Be free with your compliments, like telling your partner he is handsome.
• Avoid being overly critical and unromantic, or acting too aggressively about having sex.
• Encourage your partner in his efforts; let him know in nice ways what you find exciting.
• Sexy underwear, perfume, and a readiness to cuddle can all be terrific come-ons.

YOUR SEXUAL PROFILE

The following questionnaire looks at aspects of your personality and your mastery of sexual techniques, and assesses how likely you are to succeed in sexual relationships. There are slightly different questionnaires for each partner.

WOMAN'S QUESTIONNAIRE

1 Would you take the initiative in getting to know someone to whom you were attracted?

2 Is it easy for you to be physically demonstrative with people you like?

3 Do you often hug or kiss a lover simply to show affection?

4 Do you feel that it is just as, or more, important to to please yourself sexually as sexually satisfying your partner?

5 Do you feel comfortable with erotic episodes in movies or books?

6 Do you feel comfortable and relaxed about being seen naked?

7 Do you enjoy having your body caressed by your partner?

8 Do you know your partner's erogenous zones and where he particularly likes to be touched?

9 Do you masturbate sometimes just for enjoyment?

10 Do you often initiate sex without waiting for your partner?

11 Do you communicate your enjoyment of sex to your partner?

12 Do you sometimes make love in the daytime or with the light on?

14 Do you have oral sex with your partner, or, if not, because he doesn't want to?

15 Are you skilled in masturbating your partner to orgasm?

16 Have you tried different positions for intercourse and did you enjoy them?

17 Have you ever suggested to a sexual partner an activity that you heard or read about?

18 Would you readily agree to a new sexual activity ?

19 Do you tell your partner he is not stimulating you correctly rather than faking orgasm?

20 Are you able to tell your partner if he does something you like, or dislike, during sex?

21 Are you able to arouse your partner if he is feeling uninterested in sex?

22 Is your partner able to tell you he is not in the mood for sex without you feeling rejected?

23 Are you able to tell your partner that you are not in the mood for sex without feeling guilty?

24 If you had an erotic dream about your partner, could you tell him without feeling embarrassed?

Twenty or more yes answers points to your having a satisfactory sex life; 15 to 19 yeses means that there is room for improvement (see Having It All In Your Sex Life), and 14 or below may indicate a definite problem (see Success With Sexual Problems).

YES ☐
NO ☐

MAN'S QUESTIONNAIRE

1 Are you physically demonstrative with people without feeling unmasculine? ☐ ☐

2 Do you tend to touch people occasionally when you are talking to them? ☐ ☐

3 Do you often hug and kiss a lover simply to show affection (and not just when you feel like sex)? ☐ ☐

4 Do you allow your partner to enjoy some other men's company without being jealous? ☐ ☐

5 Are you comfortable about being naked in front of your partner? ☐ ☐

6 Can your partner initiate sex without you feeling troubled? ☐ ☐

7 Do you enjoy having your body caressed by your partner? ☐ ☐

8 Do you find leisurely foreplay a waste of time or frustrating? ☐ ☐

9 Do you communicate your enjoyment of sex to your partner? ☐ ☐

10 Are you sensitive to your partner's feelings and encourage her not to worry if she has problems? ☐ ☐

11 Can you tell your partner that you love her and not feel uncomfortable? ☐ ☐

12 Do you occasionally make love in the daytime or with the light on? ☐ ☐

13 Do you have oral sex with your partner, or if not, because she doesn't want to? ☐ ☐

14 Have you varied your lovemaking technique by trying a new position or simply having sex in a different place? ☐ ☐

15 Do you suggest to a sexual partner an activity that you fantasized, heard, or read about? ☐ ☐

16 If your partner suggested a new sexual activity, would you agree without taking it as a criticism of your ability? ☐ ☐

17 Do you know the erogenous zones of your partner's body and where she likes to be touched? ☐ ☐

18 Are you skilled in masturbating your partner to orgasm? ☐ ☐

19 Do you usually talk with a partner about her and your own likes and dislikes in lovemaking? ☐ ☐

20 Do you always make sure a woman is fully aroused before you penetrate her? ☐ ☐

21 When you have an orgasm and your partner does not, do you usually try to satisfy her by other means? ☐ ☐

22 Are you able to delay your orgasm in order to prolong intercourse? ☐ ☐

23 If you have a temporary sexual difficulty, can you discuss it freely with your partner? ☐ ☐

THE SEXUAL REPERTOIRE

Here I have set out activities that are practiced by most people. There are more bizarre practices, but these occur rarely and, as they may not be embraced wholeheartedly by both partners, I haven't included them. Your sexual experience may include some or all of the below, and if the former, you might like to widen your horizons by trying the new ones out. The lists assume the active part but, for truly satisfying experiences, partners must learn how to receive as well as give.

WHAT MEN CAN DO

- You talk warmly or sexually to your partner.
- You hold or rub your body against your partner's body.
- You kiss your partner passionately.
- You kiss with your tongues in each other's mouths.
- You fondle your partner's clothed body.
- You undress your partner and see her naked.
- You caress your partner's naked body.
- You kiss your partner's breasts and lick, suck, or gently take her nipples into your mouth.
- With your hands you explore and stroke your partner's vaginal area.
- You lick and kiss around and inside your partner's vagina.
- You bring your partner to orgasm by stimulating her clitoris and vaginal area with your hands and fingers.
- You bring your partner to orgasm by stimulating her clitoris and vaginal area with your mouth.
- You reach orgasm by intercourse in any of the following positions:
  with you on top
  lying side-by-side
  with you approaching behind
  with your partner on top
  both sitting
  both kneeling
  both standing.
- You fondle or kiss your partner's buttocks and anal area.

WHAT WOMEN CAN DO

- You use sexual terms in your conversation and speak intimately to your partner.
- You take your partner's body and hold it or rub it against yours.
- You offer him a variety of kisses.
- You engage in open-mouthed kissing with your tongues in each other's mouths.
- While he is clothed, you fondle your partner's body.
- You take off your partner's clothes and look at his naked body.
- On your partner's naked body, you bestow a variety of caresses.
- You lick or suck your partner's nipples.
- Using your hands, you explore and stroke your partner's penis and testicles.
- You lick and kiss your partner's penis and testicles.
- While stimulating his penis with your hands, you bring your partner to orgasm.
- Using your mouth on his penis, you bring your partner to orgasm.
- You reach orgasm by intercourse in the following positions:
  man-on-top
  side-by-side
  woman-on-top
  rear-entry
  sitting
  kneeling
  standing.
- You caress or kiss your partner's buttocks and anus.

The Many Varieties Of Foreplay

FOREPLAY

I can't say it often enough: satisfying lovemaking takes time, and can never take too long. Fortunately, there is a wide range of activities that lovers can indulge in that do not involve actual sexual intercourse. On rare occasions, you may be so aroused that you immediately proceed to penetration and an orgasm, but usually a couple enjoys the gradual intimacies that leisurely kissing, undressing, petting, and oral sex, among other activities, provide.

The varieties of techniques that can be used to pleasure each other can be enjoyed in their own right, or as prologues to sexual intercourse. Each stage should be savored as an integral part of lovemaking. The longer, more refined, and attentive the foreplay is, the more receptive your whole body and you will become, and the better and more magical the ultimate pleasure will be.

A MAN'S NEED FOR FOREPLAY

Contrary to popular belief, men, too, need and enjoy foreplay. It offers them the necessary stimulation to build up a good, firm erection and prepare the penis for intercourse. In fact, many cases of impotence could be prevented if foreplay was sufficiently long and exciting.

There are, however, a couple of situations where the length and type of foreplay needs to be carefully discussed, and that is when a man experiences premature ejaculation or when he has trouble maintaining an erection. In those cases, if he is undergoing therapy, he may want to keep foreplay to a minimum.

Some men see foreplay as a variety of things they have to go through in order to get their partners ready for intercourse. Others have trouble accepting bodily caresses and want to move straight on to a partner's touching their genitals. Encourage your partner to appreciate the delights foreplay offers by being enthusiastic about trying new sensual experiences so that he learns that joy in sexual activities comes in a large part from the affection expressed between you, and from the stroking, fondling, kissing, hugging, etc., that should go on.

A WOMAN'S NEED FOR FOREPLAY

A woman's body needs prolonged stimulation if she is to become fully aroused. Arousal is induced by a complex blend of mental and physical stimuli when the emotional atmosphere is sufficiently encouraging.

Some women need a particularly long time, and a considerate man must therefore wait for his partner, dominate his impulses, and hold back his reflexes. As you arouse your partner, you also will feel intense pleasure, and she will not only be more receptive but more helpful during intercourse, so that the experience becomes equally pleasurable for both of you. Men who kiss and cuddle their partners a lot, and indulge in sensitive foreplay, are much more likely to see their partners reach orgasm frequently and easily.

Don't be in a hurry to remove your partner's clothes and proceed immediately to touching her breasts and vagina. Hold her close, and keep early caresses nongenital. Concentrate on your partner. Let the resulting feelings range all over your body, and avoid thinking solely about what is happening to your penis.

UNDRESSING

Removing your clothes, and those of your partner, can be a very exciting and important part of foreplay. Undressing not only results in general arousal, but the wearing of or the removal of particular garments can strike a much more resonant chord in a susceptible lover, particularly a man.

A good lover will seek to discover which garments and their removal will act as turn-ons, and will make use of them to increase a partner's pleasure. You may have to practice removing the clothes of the other sex with one hand, without clumsiness or hold-ups, if undressing is to be truly exciting.

Nudity may become routine and boring, particularly in marriage, so some subtlety in undressing is worth retaining. Even after years of living together, undressing each other will be a highly arousing thing to do; each partner should feel more and more excited as one garment after another is removed.

WHAT A MAN FINDS EXCITING

Many men prefer a hint of nudity to complete nudity because it allows the imagination to run riot. Lovely, lacy, fine lingerie is attractive to and exciting for men, both the sight of it and its removal. Your partner may enjoy making love especially when you retain an undergarment such as a slip, stockings, garter belt, panties, bra, or camisole.

The removal of certain clothes — those that emphasize a woman's breasts, buttocks, and genitals — is almost universally a turn-on. Women who take their time about getting undressed and who "accidentally" reveal parts of themselves are certain to excite their partners. And, if a woman strips in front of her partner, this active display of herself has an impact which no man can fail to find extremely erotic. The memory of his partner taking off her clothes may prove irresistible, and he will want to recreate this scene over and over again in his mind.

WHAT A WOMAN FINDS EXCITING

Wearing lovely, lacy, fine lingerie is attractive to and exciting for women and many like to retain an undergarment such as a slip, stockings, garter belt, panties, bra, or camisole during the early stages of foreplay. Many women also like their partners occasionally to retain some of their garments during sex, though not their socks. A hint of nudity allows the imagination to run wild.

A lot of women prefer to have their partners undress them because it allows them to show off their bodies passively without being sexually overt. Other women may feel sufficiently confident to strip in front of their partners. If done with drama and artistry (something that may require a bit of enjoyable practice in front of a mirror), it will be highly erotic — mainly because the woman's role is no longer a passive one. She is actively displaying herself in an attempt to arouse her partner, and he knows this.

KISSING

A kiss is very often the first expression of love, and no matter in what other sexual activities a person may indulge, kissing may remain one of the most voluptuous caresses. The mouth is highly responsive and mobile, and can offer a great variety of sensual pleasures. Through it we are able to experience touch, taste, and smell at the same time.

Kisses can be tender, light, and lingering, or passionate, deep, burning, and even rough. Between couples who are strongly attracted to each other, it can mimic the act of intercourse; the tongue penetrates the mouth with a rhythmical intensity, as does the penis the woman's body.

There is an infinite variety to kisses, with lips closed or open, dry or moist, still or moving, explorative or quietly tender. What lends variety to kissing, too, is that it can be done to any part of the body. It should not be restricted to mouth-to-mouth contact; kissing should be used on every crease and crevice. Kissing your lover's erogenous zones, particularly the genital parts, can be the most intimate and stimulating part of foreplay, and here kisses can result in the most profound reactions. For some people, kissing is a necessary accompaniment to orgasm and lends passion and depth to their climaxes.

Heightened sexual response
A kiss can be highly arousing. A woman can feel it in the breasts and genital area, and often by itself, it can result in orgasm.

WHAT A MAN LIKES

Although the notion persists in a few men that kissing may be a sign of weakness, the vast majority enjoy the physical closeness and body contact that it brings. Few men, however, would be content to stop at kissing, especially if there was any possibility of intercourse, and often kisses that are meant affectionately without further promise can be misunderstood by them as an invitation to greater intimacy.

Men love to be kissed passionately, and you will be almost certain to arouse your partner by kissing and caressing certain areas such as the back of his neck, his ears, and eyelids. Use deep, sensuous kisses to stimulate his lips, tongue, and the inside of his mouth. Flick your tongue in and out of his mouth and try to have your tongues touching.

Gentle biting and nibbling can be highly erotic as well, but it's best to avoid "love bites" on the genitals, which are highly sensitive and may be damaged or caused excessive pain. While some men particularly enjoy having their nipples kissed and sucked, most men love best to have their penises kissed (see also Performing Fellatio, p. 82).

WHAT A WOMAN LIKES

Women enjoy kissing very much, and most complain that they don't get enough of it — too many men proceed to genital touching far too soon. Women enjoy a gradual progression to the genitals, and like having their ears, necks, shoulders, breasts, stomachs, inner thighs, knees, and feet kissed along the way. Women use kissing as a way of initiating sex and stimulating interest in their partners.

Simple kisses on the lips can be delicious, but many women enjoy deep tongue-to-tongue kisses and hard, prolonged kisses on the lips. You will be almost certain to arouse your partner by kissing and caressing certain areas such as the back of her neck, her hair, ears, cheeks, and eyelids. Use deep, sensuous kisses to stimulate your partner's lips and tongue, and the inside of her mouth. Flick your tongue in and out of her mouth and try to have your tongues touching.

Gentle biting and nibbling can be highly erotic as well, but it's best to avoid "love bites" on the genitals, which are highly sensitive and may be damaged or caused excessive pain, and on the breasts, where gentle sucking is more widely preferred. Some women can even reach orgasm this way. And for many women, kissing can be an end in itself.

EROGENOUS ZONES

Discovering and exploring your partner's erogenous zones should be loving, caring, and thoughtful, not simply mechanical. Every woman should try to discover as much as possible about her man's body, and every man should experiment to find out what exactly will please his partner. Couples should learn to excite each other slowly but surely, and gradually find out which certain parts of the body will provide pleasure and stimulation when touched.

As you kiss and stroke various parts of your partner's body, he or she should let you know immediately what effect your touch has, and you should always express the rising excitement that you feel. Mutual feedback is needed.

For both men and women, stimulation of the erogenous zones begins with the hands and fingers, but, of course, all these areas respond even more intensely to touches from the mouth, lips, and tongue. In addition to gentle stroking, patting, and rubbing, occasional gentle slaps should be used also to bring variety to sensation and lovemaking techniques. Men will also enjoy their partners using their breasts and nipples to stroke and caress them; women find the most potent touch is from the penis, particularly the glans penis, which to them is a miracle of softness and hardness.

DISCOVERING A MAN'S EROGENOUS ZONES

Like those erogenous zones enjoyed by women such as the lips, any area of the face, and the fingertips, there are certain general areas of a man's body which are very pleasurable for him when touched, such as the shoulders, the palms of the hands, the back, the chest, and the nipples. Stroking and sucking your partner's nipples provides pleasure and they will become erect, a sign of arousal.

The whole of a man's genital area responds to the slightest touch, and within this area there are many specific points to be explored. The area just behind the root of the penis, between the penis and the anus, that overlies the prostate gland, can be exceptionally sensitive to touch, both in arousal and in reaching orgasm. The testicles are extremely sensitive and must be handled gently, as excessive or clumsy handling can be painful. But unquestionably, the penis is a man's most sensitive erogenous zone, and the place where he feels the most intense sensations and where pleasure is concentrated. The entire shaft of the penis is very sensitive, but the glans at the tip is particularly rich in nerve endings, especially on its crown, and it will react very quickly to the slightest stimulation. The frenulum, too, is extremely sensitive in all men, as is the area lying just behind the opening.

The buttocks are a sexually arousable area, and most men find pleasure in having their buttocks caressed; some men also like having them gently slapped or spanked. There are also a lot of erotic nerve endings around the anus and this area, too, is highly sensitive to caresses of all types.

DISCOVERING A WOMAN'S EROGENOUS ZONES

In contrast with a man, the whole of a woman's skin is an erogenous zone and all of it will respond to touches, caresses, and kisses. However, there are certain areas where stimulation results in more intense arousal. These erogenous zones vary from woman to woman, and a man must find out where they are, and while making love, should stimulate them in gentle and personal ways.

GENERAL BODY AREAS

A woman's face, for instance, has several erogenous zones including her hairline, forehead, temples, eyebrows, eyelids, and cheeks. In general, women prefer light caresses that barely touch their faces. The mouth for most women is one of their most erogenous zones, and it can be stimulated readily with fingertip touching and kisses. Stimulating a woman's mouth, however, can set her whole body alight, and has a direct effect in arousing her genital organs. On the other hand, erogenous stimulation of any other part of a woman's body often produces a reaction in her mouth, in her breasts, and in her genital organs as well.

The earlobes are extremely sensitive to stimulation and can be caressed gently, but some women have such a violent reaction to their lobes being touched that they even can have an orgasm after such a simple caress. The neck, particularly at the back, is a very sensitive area, as is the part just down the sides. A woman's acceptance of long kisses on the neck usually means that she is ready to accept kisses elsewhere. The arms, the armpits, the hands and the back, the hips and the entire lower abdomen can be stimulated erotically by an attentive lover.

An extremely sensitive zone is the area around the navel. Most women relish caresses with the fingertips, lips, or penis over the whole length of their legs and particularly on the inner side of the thighs.

THE MOST RESPONSIVE SITES

For most women the breasts are highly erotic and play a vital part in sexual excitement. Sucking, nibbling, licking, stroking, and gentle squeezing will cause the nipples to become erect, a certain sign of arousal. However, women do differ greatly in their reactions to breast stimulation so it's important to find out what exactly she likes and doesn't like.

The most erogenous area of a woman's body includes the perineum, an area of skin between the vagina and the anus. If you put your whole hand on this area, with the outer lips of the vagina closed, and press hard or massage, a woman can be aroused very quickly because of the dense network of nerve endings.

Both the inner and outer lips of the perineal area are extremely rich in nerve endings also, and are a highly erogenous zone in all sexually experienced women. The inner lips, however, are much more sensitive than the outer ones — especially if stroked along their inner surfaces along the cleft of the vulva. If you press both lips together and firmly massage with your fingers all the sensitive parts of the vulva, high excitement should result. The clitoris is the most sexually sensitive part of a woman's body, and the easiest part to stimulate if a man can only learn to do it gently and skillfully without undue haste. Stimulation of the clitoris with the tip of the erect penis is a particularly pleasurable sensation to many women.

As with the mouth, the entrance to the vagina is rich in nerve endings and reacts intensely to all sorts of caresses — the ultimate being from the glans penis — but it can be ecstatic for some women to be caressed there by a man's lips and his tongue.

The buttocks are another erogenous zone and their many nerve endings are easily stimulated by patting, rubbing, or gentle slaps.

PINPOINTING EROGENOUS ZONES

Certain areas of the body, especially parts of the skin, are particularly sensitive sexually. These areas are called erogenous zones. Their sensitivity is due to their rich supply of sensory nerve endings, which pick up touch. In a sexual situation, touch stimuli become sexual stimuli. Where the emotional component is very high, touch of almost any part of the body can become a sexual stimulus and this is why almost any part of the skin can be an erogenous zone, if it is touched by a sexually attractive and desirable partner. The areas of the body where a dry surface meets a moist surface usually contain large quantities of sensitive nerves, and react very quickly to touch.

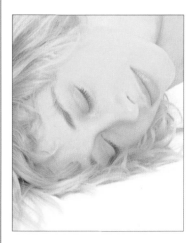

Lips
A woman's, or a man's, lips are obvious erogenous zones that respond to touch, kissing, or licking.

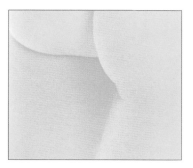

Thighs
The inner thigh, a very sensitive area, can be source of erotic pleasure when stroked, licked, or kissed.

Body
The entire body, and particularly the skin, can become one large erogenous zone.

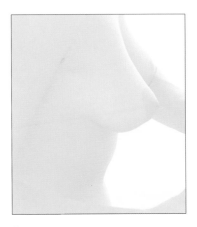

Breasts
A woman's breasts are very sexually sensitive — gentle or slightly rougher fondling and squeezing, and caressing of the nipples can be arousing.

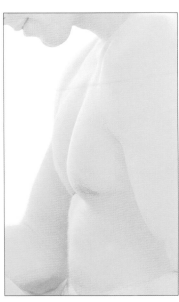

Chest
A man's chest, and his nipples as well, respond to kissing and caressing.

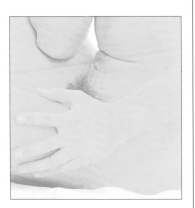

Genitals
Both partners' genitals contain the largest number of sensory nerve endings, and stimulation of these areas produces quick and powerful sexual feelings.

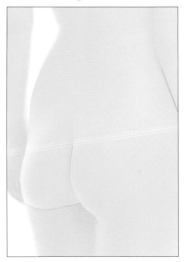

Buttocks
The buttocks, visual symbols of sensuality, contain many nerve endings and are definite erogenous zones.

PETTING

Whether sexual intercourse is on the agenda or not, a man's generalized kissing and cuddling will lead eventually to his touching, caressing, and kissing a woman's breasts, nipples, and clitoris, and a woman will be encouraged to do the same for a man's scrotum and penis. Petting, or love play using fingers, has a value that is more than just being romantic. It is vital to the escalating spiral of sexual excitement necessary for satisfying sexual intercourse.

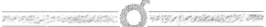

WHAT A MAN LIKES

Kissing should lead into and blend with caresses over the man's whole body. Passionate kissing, sucking, and stroking are all pleasurable. Vivid sensations can be produced in a man, too, by slowly and seductively rubbing your hands or other body parts on his bare skin.

A man is easily turned on by having his genitals stimulated (though it is in a woman's interest to prolong foreplay and delay genital caresses until nearer to penetration), and many men also enjoy having their buttocks stroked or kneaded. Some men will enjoy gentle smacking. Many men also enjoy having their scrotums and testes held, and sometimes squeezed. The crescendo reached in such ascending sexual activity can frequently bring a man to orgasm without penetrative sex ever taking place.

Petting is extremely potent. Sexual excitement begins with some stimulus that orders the pituitary gland in the brain to send out a hormone that travels through the bloodstream to stimulate the testicles into releasing more hormones, and this makes a man feel sexy and aroused. The hormones themselves push the hypothalmus into producing more of its hormone. This process is an escalating spiral in which the sexier a man feels, the more sexy he will feel. It is in a woman's interest to maintain this high level of arousal.

WHAT A WOMAN LIKES

One of the reasons why petting is so powerful and so enjoyed by women is that it arouses and relaxes them, and prepares them for attempting intercourse. For women, intercourse is only welcome when they feel ready and have had enough stimulation so that the vagina lubricates and unfolds in readiness to receive the penis. Without the chance to build up the level of sex hormones through kissing, caressing, and, most importantly, petting, intercourse can be very uncomfortable for a woman.

The majority of men underestimate how long this takes since their own erections occur much more quickly.

Kissing should lead into and blend with caresses over her entire body. Most women prefer initial caresses to be in areas other than the breasts and genitals, but once they have begun to feel aroused, they do enjoy having their breasts and bottoms stimulated. Breasts, however, need careful stroking until a woman is more highly aroused, then more passionate kissing, sucking, and stroking will be pleasurable. Most women like their buttocks caressed and squeezed, and some will enjoy gentle smacking. Only when a woman is sufficiently aroused does she want her partner to move on to genital caresses (see page 78). Women are not universal in their tastes but most prefer initial genital caresses to be gentle, with harder, more vigorous movements as they near orgasm.

MASSAGE

I believe that mastering the techniques of sexual and nonsexual touching is very important to a satisfactory sexual relationship. For people who already enjoy a good sex life, massage can enhance enjoyment; for most of us, there is plenty of room for improvement.

Massage is important because not only does it have the general effect of relaxing you and giving you the opportunity to really think about and enjoy touching, but it allows you to focus your senses acutely and deeply on the responses aroused in your body, and in this way increases your sex drive. During massage some people experience this "sensate focusing" for the first time.

Massage can be particularly important for women because it can have exactly the same effect as kissing, caressing, and other forms of foreplay, in that it allows a woman's sex hormones to build up and to arouse and prepare her body for intercourse. It is helpful also for men who have difficulty in arousal or suffer from impotence (see also Success With Your Sexual Problems).

One of the aims of massage is to give you the opportunity to discover for yourself what gives you pleasure, and you should approach it with a completely open mind. Men and women are often surprised how sexy it feels to have certain parts of their bodies caressed, although they had never thought of them as remotely erotic.

— GETTING THE MAXIMUM PLEASURE —

Getting to know every inch of your lover's body is among the most pleasurable shared experiences, and it is worth taking the time and trouble to set the scene properly. You should alternate between being the passive or pleasure-giving partner. Choose a time when you won't be interrupted, and a place that is warm and private. Soft lighting and background music also can contribute. You can use a bed that isn't too soft, or the floor with sufficient cushions.

Both partners should adopt comfortable positions and should be undressed to get the maximum benefit. The person giving the massage should make certain his or her hands are warm and preferably oiled. If you are the pleasure-giving partner, concentrate on what you are doing and how your partner is responding. If it is your turn to be on the receiving end, lie back and enjoy every minute.

Start with a gentle, exploratory massage going over all parts of your partner's body except the genitals and breasts, as this will make the process much more sensual and relaxed. Of course, you can, if you like, go on to touching the breasts and genitals, and this may prove so arousing that sexual intercourse or an orgasm cannot be avoided.

MASSAGE TECHNIQUES

Massage depends on using the hands, thumbs, and fingers to apply rhythmical pressure to your partner's body. There are various techniques, and a variety of these should be used for the maximum pleasure. The most important things are to keep up a slow, steady rhythm with sufficient pressure, and to make sure your hands glide smoothly over your partner's body as in effleurage, shown below.

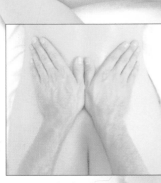

Start with the thumbs on either side of the spine and your fingers pointing toward the head.

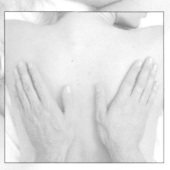

Work your way up from the lower back, stroking firmly and keeping your hands relaxed.

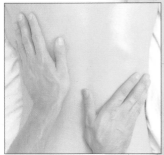

Use alternating strokes: one hand strokes firmly upward, the other glides down.

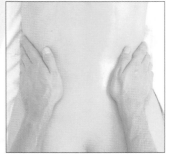

Fan your hands out over the lower back; press on the spinal muscles on either side.

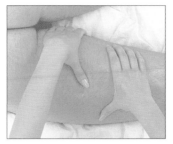

Kneading
Useful on fleshy areas such as the hips and thighs, the effect can be changed by varying the depth and speed — slow and deep or fast and superficial. Lift, squeeze, and roll the flesh between the thumb and fingers of one hand and glide it toward the other hand.

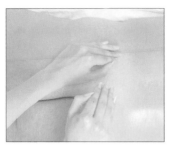

Cupping
Quick, light movements are stimulating and refreshing to the skin. Strike the body lightly with alternate hands, keeping your thumbs tucked in and the fingers together. As your hands touch the body they should make a hollow popping sound.

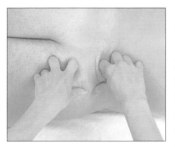

Knuckling
Curl your fingers into loose fists, keeping the middle of your fingers pressed against the skin, and make small circling movements. A rippling effect is produced, which is pleasant on the shoulders, chest, palms, and soles.

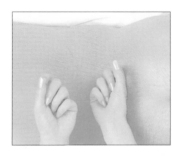

Pummeling
Percussive movements, which are brisk and bouncy, should be used on fleshy, muscular areas. With the hands in loose fists, lightly bounce the sides of the hands alternately against the skin. Use these movements at the end of a massage to rouse your partner.

MASSAGING AIDS

Various scented oils are available that leave the skin soft and smooth, and add to the occasion with their fragrance. Apply the oil sparingly to your hands and then to the body parts you will be massaging. Feathers, fabric, and other soft textures can be rubbed against the skin.

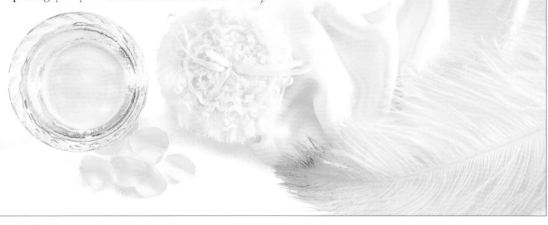

MASSAGE: WHAT A MAN CAN DO

When a man slowly and gently caresses his partner, he reassures her of his love for her and her body. A woman has many erotic areas, and a man should take time over them, stroking gently with a light pressure and some circular movements to elicit strong, pleasurable sensations. Her head and neck, lips, mouth, and earlobes are highly sensitive, as are her breasts, genital area, belly, and buttocks.

Touch her face
Trace your partner's lips and face with gentle strokes. The mouth, jawline, neck, and ears are all highly sensitive and receptive of touch.

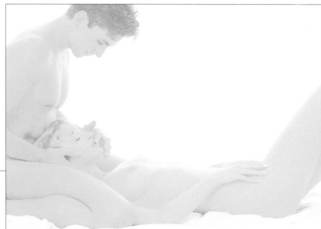

Stroke her chest
Place your hands over your partner's breastbone and glide them steadily downward; then curve outward.

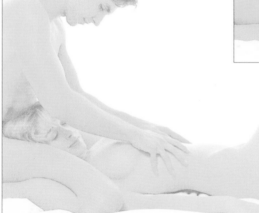

Softly murmur
endearments to make
your partner feel
desirable

Caress her breasts
Caress your partner's breasts,
cupping your hands and fingers
softly around the sides and
underneath, and circling her
nipples with light strokes.

Let your partner lean
against your chest in
a comfortable
position

Skin-to-skin
contact will
make the
experience more
sensuous

MASSAGE: WHAT A WOMAN CAN DO

In addition to gentle stroking and caressing with your hands, a sensual massage can include other means of stimulation such as kissing, licking, soft blowing, and brushing your partner's body with your breasts or hair. You can sit, kneel beside him, or straddle him, so that he can feel the warmth of your inner thighs, producing a heightened response. You can use your full hands, fingertips, just your thumbs, or the heels of the hands. Either gently knead and rub his back and upper body with long, rhythmic strokes, or run your fingers lightly and tantalizingly up and down the sides of his back. Or you can massage a different region, such as his inner thighs, buttocks, or feet, all of which are highly erogenous and heighten your partner's pleasure.

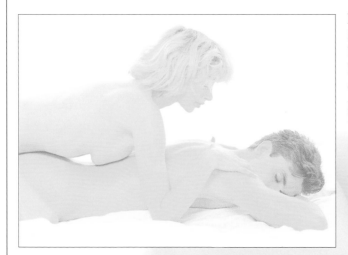

Massage his back
Straddling your partner, begin by resting your hands on his body for a few moments to establish body contact, and then proceed to lightly massage his back and upper body.

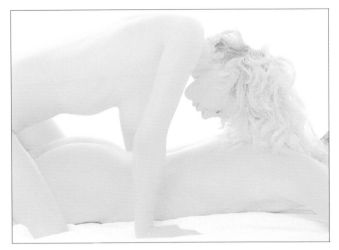

Stroke his back with your hair
Brush your partner's back gently with your hair or breasts, keeping your weight off him by supporting yourself with your hands or elbows.

Press your body against his to increase the intimacy

Kiss his neck
Draping one leg or arm across his body, kiss your partner's neck, blow softly in his ear, and stroke his neck and shoulders with your hands.

MASTURBATION

The majority of both men and women come to know about their own sexuality through masturbation, which usually starts around age 10 or 11. Of course, boys and girls do play with themselves long before this, particularly boys, who may grasp their penises in their first year of life, but only because it is an appendage that juts out from the rest of them.

As a pleasurable sensation, though not a sexual one, children fondle themselves around the age of 3 and 4, and may explore each other around the ages of 5 and 6, but it is not until adolescence has started and male and female sex hormones are being produced, that masturbation for sexual pleasure starts. Ten or 11 would be the earliest, but it can start much later in some people, so that for many, masturbation is not experienced until the late teens or early 20s.

It is only through personal experimentation that people come to understand their preferences and develop techniques that they find most pleasing. But it is essential that these preferences are expressed to a partner, and that the techniques are candidly shared.

In most people, autoerotic experience is highly private and masturbation is one of the most difficult of all topics for couples to discuss. Perhaps religious orientation forbids it, or it still may be an area they feel unable to discuss because it is so highly private. Many people find masturbation a difficult subject to approach because they think they have to share what they actually do. This isn't at all necessary, but you should try to share with your partner how you feel.

Autoeroticism, of course, is not limited to self-stimulation of the genital organs; there are many other experiences in life that are autoerotic, such as taking a long, luxurious, sensuous bath, or simply feeling the wind in your hair and the sun on your skin. Don't limit your view of autoeroticism entirely to sex; give yourself permission to be stimulated by the many naturally occurring, everyday experiences like a crisp, sunny winter morning, a walk along the beach on a fine day, or swimming in the sea or a pool.

ATTITUDES TOWARD MASTURBATION

Many people think of masturbation as unnatural and disgusting and a complete waste of time, and don't understand why anybody does it and are quite unsympathetic to the view that people might continue to do it even though they have sexual partners. The majority of men, though they may keep their feelings to themselves, don't agree.

For most people, once it is faced, masturbation in front of, or with a partner, and particularly if it is mutual, can be an extremely enjoyable and exciting way of making love, especially if it comes at the end of an extended period of foreplay. Differences in attitudes can be ironed out only if you are candid with your partner and voice your feelings about masturbation. You may get a shock: you may find that you are both attracted to the idea.

There are many myths about masturbation, all of them untrue, but it is important for everyone to realize that masturbation cannot cause any trouble for anyone unless it is against one's own moral sanctions. It should be seen as an excellent opportunity for self-education. Your attitude to it should be open and comfortable; it should never end up leaving impressions of hurriedness, guilt, or secretiveness about sex. More importantly, masturbation can lead to intense orgasms, and it is the one way to develop sexual comfort, security, and self-esteem.

Above all, masturbation is not something that means sex with your partner is not as good as it should be, or even that your partner cannot stimulate your genital organs in the way that you have become accustomed to. Many partners have their best sexual experiences when masturbation or mutual masturbation is engaged in prior to or during sexual intercourse.

WHAT A MAN LIKES

Male masturbation always has been a secret from which women have been excluded. Even within marriage, few women are given the opportunity to witness it. But without knowledge of how your partner gives himself pleasure, it is difficult for you to do so. There is no better way to learn than to look and talk.

A man's sexual focus is the head of his penis; this is in marked contrast to women, who have a greater range of sensation-producing apparatus. (In addition to the high level of sexual response concentrated on the clitoral shaft and glans, women can be excited by stimulation of the labia, the opening into the vagina, and the vagina itself.) Touching the scrotal sac and the testes is not as exciting for men as stimulation of the labial area or the vaginal entrance is for women.

A man concentrates his efforts on the glans and frenulum, since the shaft is relatively insensitive and serves to let his hand move up and down rhythmically.

WHAT A WOMAN LIKES

The easiest way for a man to find out how a woman likes to be stimulated, and how much stimulation is necessary, is to study how women masturbate. Some women, especially those who may have guilty feelings about self-pleasuring, however, prefer to be masturbated by their partners. Some women do it at particular times, such as while menstruating, and keep it secret from their partners. Others, especially more "liberated" women, indulge in it routinely as a way of relieving sexual tension. And because direct and continued genital stimulation is so necessary to a woman's orgasm, some women use self-masturbation as a way of guaranteeing that they reach a climax while having intercourse.

In fact, since only about 30 percent of women experience a climax with intercourse but over 80 percent achieve orgasm with masturbation, orgasm through masturbation, rather than intercourse, should be regarded as the normal experience.

——— MASTURBATION CAN BE FUN ———

Masturbation is an option, a way of mutually enhancing a couple's sexual enjoyment. Masturbation is generally helpful to sexuality in all areas of your life. That doesn't mean to say that if you don't masturbate you're abnormal; you're not inadequate or deficient.

Remember also that masturbation does not mean anything good or bad about your marital sex; in fact, there is some evidence that shows that people who masturbate without guilt are able to be freer in expressing their sexuality, more aware of the nature of their own individual sexual response, and therefore, enjoy sex more than those who are guilt-ridden. Moreover, masturbation is a worthwhile alternative to intercourse when a woman is very pregnant or just had a baby, or if she is recovering from gynecological surgery; or when a man cannot get an erection.

CAN A MAN MASTURBATE TOO MUCH?

Men commonly report masturbatory frequency ranging from once a month to two or three times a day. Nearly every man is concerned about the supposed mental effects of excessive masturbation, but every man considers excessive levels of masturbation to consist of a higher frequency than his own personal practice. A man who masturbates once a month sees once or twice a week as excessive, with mental illness as a quite possible complication of such frequency. A man who masturbates two or three times a day thinks five or six times a day is excessive, and might lead to a case of nerves. No man, however, has the slightest fear that his particular masturbatory pattern is excessive, regardless of frequency.

There is no medically accepted standard defining excessive masturbation, and there is no medical evidence that masturbation, regardless of frequency, leads to any form of mental illness. In fact, the case may be that men masturbate too little — both in time spent and in number of occasions. More pleasure, more sensuality, and more control can be positive results of masturbatory activity.

CAN A WOMAN MASTURBATE TOO MUCH?

For most women, masturbation is the introduction to sex. Few women have a clear idea of their own sexual anatomy, and so wouldn't know where they like being stimulated unless they'd masturbated. Masturbation helps a girl to know how she functions sexually, and it helps her to form preferences. It almost certainly gives her the first orgasm.

Women often can find it harder achieving orgasm than men, and the ability to discover what feels good and exciting, what arouses them, and what makes them less inhibited, less fearful, and more willing to let go, is most often discovered through masturbation. Having once achieved orgasm by this means, it becomes easier to repeat.

Masturbation is important, too, for older women — those with partners and those without. It increases lubrication and diminishes vaginal pain due to dryness. Whether masturbation has been continual, or whether it is taken up again on the loss of a partner, it is an ideal sexual activity — an easy way to orgasm — and one that is guaranteed to prolong your sexually active life.

WHAT MEN DO

It is only through personal experimentation that each man discovers how best he likes to be stimulated. Some men use the lightest touch on the upper surface of the penis; some use strong, gripping, and stroking movements over the whole organ that for many other individuals would be quite objectionable if not painful. Frequently, men prefer stimulation of the glans alone, either confining manipulation to the surface of the penis on or near the frenulum, or pulling to stimulate the entire glans area. Most men, however, manipulate the shaft of the penis with stroking movements that encompass the entire organ; rapidity, length of movement, and tightness vary from man to man.

Many men masturbate incorrectly; they try to get it done quickly and much of their technique and timing is wrong. This may lead to problems later on because many men associate masturbation and ejaculation with getting rid of tension quickly.

As ejaculation approaches, most men increase their actions until they are stroking the penile shaft as rapidly as possible. During ejaculation, most men either ease completely or markedly slow the movements along the penile shaft. This is because the glans is quite sensitive immediately after ejaculation. (This situation is rarely appreciated by women, who often have completely different preferences as regards stimulation. See right.) It can be distressing for her partner if a woman continues active manual stroking or pelvic thrusting immediately subsequent to ejaculation.

Some men find using a lubricant on their hands can reduce friction and enhance their pleasure. Petroleum jelly, hand or body lotions, and massage oils all have their adherents, and all contribute toward making the experience more pleasurable.

WHAT WOMEN DO

No two women masturbate in the same way, although they rarely manipulate the glans of the clitoris directly, since it often becomes extremely sensitive to touch or pressure. This is particularly so immediately after orgasm, and care has to be taken to avoid direct contact with the glans unless renewed stimulation is desired. Some women move their bodies to feel sensuous, others lie still and only let their hands work.

Most women who manipulate the clitoris do so through the shaft, manipulating the right side if right-handed and vice versa. Many women change sides; concentrated manipulation can cause numbness if too much pressure is applied to any one area. Changing sides restores sensitivity while stimulation remains unbroken.

Very few women concentrate on the clitoral body itself; most stimulate the mons area in general. Indeed, the entire perineal area becomes extremely sensitive to touch; the labia minora may be as important as the clitoris or mons as a source of erotic arousal.

During masturbation, most women manipulate the shaft of the clitoris continuously throughout the whole experience right up to orgasm and through it without a break. It is useful to know that this is the opposite of the usual man's reaction to orgasm, which is to stop rapid pelvic thrusting; stopping clitoral stimulation can account for the lack of a satisfactory female orgasm during intercourse.

Unlike a man, a woman who masturbates often is not content with one single orgasm but may enjoy several subsequent orgasms until fatigue intervenes.

Some techniques of masturbation, like rolling on an object or climaxing through the clenching of the perineal muscles, are difficult to integrate with sexual intercourse, and a woman may need to rethink or adjust her practices when a partner is involved.

STIMULATING A WOMAN

The clitoris is delicate and sensitive and a gentle approach is best. Do not use direct pressure unless your partner likes it. Most women find indirect pressure more comfortable and stimulating. Your fingers must be well lubricated, so use vaginal fluid, saliva, or jellies to minimize irritation.

To provide the most satisfying sensations over the entire clitoral area, use the whole hand — all the fingers, the palm, and the heel of the hand — rather than just one or two fingers. There are two major types of movement, circular and vibratory.

For circular movements, place your hand over the clitoral area. Apply light pressure with your palm or fingers, moving them gently around and around.

Move your hand so that the heel is right over the clitoris at the top of the vulva and is resting partly on the pubic bone on either side, where you can press firmly as you rub.

Or, you can press gently with your hand, palm downward over the pubic mound so that your fingers overhang the clitoris, and make firm, circular movements.

For vibratory movements, cup your hand over the pubic area and vibrate it rapidly, brushing your fingers to and fro across the clitoris. Then, keeping your hand still, put a finger on each side of the vaginal lips and vibrate them from side to side. Pressing firmly through the fleshy folds, rub on each side of the inner vaginal lips at the base of the clitoris.

Most women also enjoy being penetrated by a finger while their clitoris is being stimulated. Make sure your fingernail is short and straight before slipping your middle finger into the vagina, keeping your other fingers bent forward so that the knuckles continue to press against the clitoris. You can move your finger in and out gently, pressing on the front wall of the vagina. Alternatively, rub the tip of your penis against the clitoris.

Placing your hand over your partner's entire perineum or vaginal area, while applying light pressure and circular movements, will increase her arousal

When your partner is sufficiently lubricated, insert your finger into her vagina and move it gently in and out, maintaining contact with the clitoris

Hold the penis close to the head to ensure good stimulation of the shaft of the penis, as well as the glans and frenulum

Your partner may want to control the rhythm. With his hand over yours, grasp the penis firmly, though gently, and move your hand rhythmically up and down the shaft, either quickly or slowly as your partner wishes

STIMULATING A MAN

To be a good lover, knowing how to stimulate the penis is one of the most valuable skills a woman can possess. Older men especially may need direct stimulation to reach erection, but men of all ages enjoy the sensations they receive from manipulation. You can use these techniques both as an adjunct to, and as a replacement for, intercourse. Vary your approach as much as you like, perhaps rolling the penis between your palms, gently stroking it with your fingers, alternately squeezing and letting it go, brushing your fingertips against the frenulum or caressing the penis between your breasts.

As a way of enhancing his sensations, and especially if your partner has erection difficulties, use a lubricant (see page 85).

Begin by positioning yourself on your partner's appropriate side — right if you are right-handed, left if you are left-handed. Grip his penis firmly with your thumb pointing toward his navel. Move your hand up and down on the penis in a regular rhythm, keeping your grip steady and the firmest pressure on the sensitive area on the uppermost side of the erect penis. Experiment with long and short strokes. A slow rhythm prolongs pleasure while a speeded-up one intensifies pleasure and will bring him to orgasm sooner.

Climax is imminent when your partner's muscles, especially those in his thighs, tense up and his breathing becomes more rapid. The testes will be drawn up to his body and may be swollen. The head of the penis will darken in color and increase slightly in size. One or two drops of preejaculatory fluid may ooze from the tip of his penis.

Your partner will want you to continue stimulation until ejaculation is completely over and his tension relaxes. Then stop stroking the penis since it usually feels very sensitive. Most men will want you to desist from further genital caresses for a while.

ORAL SEX

Fellatio, sucking or otherwise stimulating a penis with the mouth, with or without ejaculation, is almost always the most powerful way of arousing a man, and all find it intensely exciting.

The mouth appears to men to be similar to, but more exciting than, a vagina, particularly because the tongue is actively used to stimulate. In fact, the mouth is exceptionally well designed for sexual pleasure and is capable of a broad range of activities such as stroking, kissing, licking, probing, and penetrating. The mouth is also the recipient of a wide variety of sensations including the many tastes and scents of a lover's body parts.

Cunnilingus, using the tongue and mouth to lick and nuzzle the clitoris and vaginal area, is highly arousing to a great many women. The tongue is softer than the fingers so it provides gentler and more varied stimulation. Most men are willing, if not always eager, to perform cunnilingus on their partners.

There is no doubt that oral sex is intensely intimate and that it demands a level of trust rarely found elsewhere in lovemaking; for one thing, the acts can be extremely painful if care isn't taken. This intimacy contributes to the participants' satisfaction since it implies total acceptance of each other. To some people, it is the ultimate expression of love.

MAKING IT FUN

Fear of ejaculate in the mouth will be minimized if partners agree beforehand on what is to be done. If ejaculation in the mouth is to be avoided, the man should signal and withdraw in time so that his partner can continue with manual stimulation. Fear of choking is easily dealt with by the woman controlling how much of the penis she takes into her mouth, or by encircling the base of the penis with her hand to hold back his thrusting.

Worry about body odors can be dispelled by daily bathing — afterward the healthy odor of sexual arousal will prove pleasant and exciting. A woman should not try to disguise her natural smells or flavors with sprays or deodorants, which can prove intrusive, and anyway, most men find the acid taste of vaginal juices pleasant.

Never get so carried away during sex play that you bite the sex organs. Don't blow into your lover's genitals, as this can be dangerous, and never indulge in oral sex if you have a cold sore or genital infection. It is also a good idea not to indulge in oral sex with a casual partner whose sexual history is unknown to you. There is some evidence that the AIDS virus can be transmitted this way.

PERFORMING CUNNILINGUS

While some men perform cunnilingus because they find it intensely exciting, others do it more to please their partners. If you are in the latter group, you should never let your partner think you find it a chore. That is a sure turn-off. Concentrate instead on the certain knowledge that you will be giving her maximum pleasure. Remember, too, to use your hands to caress her breasts, thighs, and buttocks at the same time.

If your partner seems to be a bit reluctant, reassure her about how nice the experience is, especially if you think she is worried about her genitals tasting or smelling bad. You shouldn't have trouble sympathizing with her if you bear in mind that you have odors and tastes, too.

HOW TO PLEASURE HER

Women need direct stimulation in order to reach orgasm, so the most important thing a man can do for his partner sexually is to learn the areas, pressures, and rhythms that excite her most. The clitoris is the most sensitive part of a woman's anatomy and it may easily become intensely tender. It is often better initially to direct your attentions to the labia minora and the vaginal entrance.

Begin by kissing and licking her lower belly and the insides of her thighs, working down to her pubic mound. Then move your tongue over the genital area, flicking it along the fleshy folds up to the clitoris. Try thrusting your tongue in and out of your partner's vagina to see if she likes it.

Separate the vaginal lips with your hands and then, using your tongue, gently probe her clitoris — first nuzzle and suck it, and then vibrate your tongue rapidly against it. With sufficient stimulation, your partner should be able to reach orgasm easily. Once she has climaxed, she will probably prefer not to be stimulated further for some time.

It is important to take care with your teeth. Keep them protected by your lips and be careful not to graze or bite the sex organs; this can be extremely painful. Make sure, too, that your fingernails are not too long.

Work your way down her abdomen, kissing and licking her skin

PERFORMING FELLATIO

Find a comfortable position; it is relaxing for your partner if he lies down, but you can kneel down in front of him while he stands or sits in a chair. He should always be immaculately clean. You can bathe together or wash him yourself, making this into more foreplay. All the time you perform fellatio, caress the rest of his body with your hands to make it really exciting for him.

You can begin by kissing and licking his penis; then, holding the shaft in one hand, swirl your tongue gently around the tip. Stimulate the tip with your tongue and push the tip of your tongue into the slit. Next, explore the shaft, running your tongue around the ridge where it meets the head, and vibrate your tongue gently against the frenulum.

When you feel ready to take his penis into your mouth, cover your teeth with your lips and take in the whole head of the penis. With your teeth well apart, move your mouth up and down, letting your partner guide your rhythm with his hands on your head. Maintain a steady rhythm and firm pressure. Make certain you don't bend the penis too far down when sucking; this can be painful. The penis should always point upward.

Gradually increase your speed until he is about to climax. Then, if you don't want him to ejaculate in your mouth, withdraw and bring him to orgasm with your hand, or switch to intercourse.

As you come to enjoy fellatio, you can experiment with other sensations. Try whirling your tongue around while the penis is deep in your mouth, push the penis in and out of your mouth, or suck on it. Remember, too, the scrotum is quite sensitive, so you can use your tongue and mouth there as well.

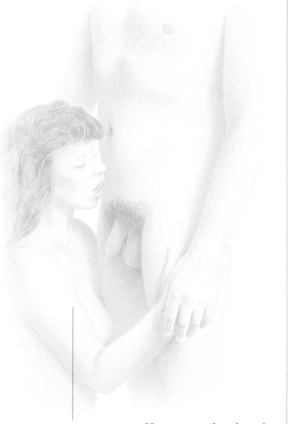

A woman can begin by kissing and caressing her partner's abdomen, thighs, and buttocks, as well as the penis and scrotum

Keeping one hand on the penile shaft or scrotum, a woman can use her lips and tongue to stimulate the head of the penis

ANAL STIMULATION

For many people, the anus and its surrounding area are very sensitive sexually, and for some it is their most erogenous zone. The anal region is well supplied with nerves that follow a similar pathway to the nerves supplying the penis and vagina. Anal stimulation, therefore, gives deep feelings of sexual pleasure unobtainable in other ways, and adds variety to lovemaking. Orgasm that occurs along with anal penetration is said to be exceptionally exquisite.

The simplest form of anal stimulation is merely touching your partner's anus during intercourse or oral sex. This is an activity known as "postillionage." More sensation can be produced by gently inserting a finger into the rectum. When doing this, lubricate your finger first, and make sure your nail isn't jagged. Never do this if you have any infection on your finger or hand.

Another technique, gluteal sex, involves the man using the crease of the woman's buttocks as an alternative to the vagina. If the woman contracts her gluteal muscles and rotates her pelvis, the man can thrust into there and reach orgasm this way.

Anal penetration carries with it the risk of AIDS, and if performed over a long time, can lead to stretching of the anal sphincter, which could lead to incontinence. However, the illicit overtones of the act (it is illegal in many parts of the world), the dominant and submissive qualities inherent in it, and the particular sensations it inspires are, to its practitioners, alluring and attractive reasons for indulging in it, and quite a few heterosexuals do.

STIMULATING A MAN

The prostate gland and rectum, when stimulated, can provide intense sensations, and this is a useful technique, especially when a man's virility is flagging. Making certain your finger, or fingers, are well lubricated (lack of a lubricant will cause very uncomfortable sensations), insert them about two inches into the rectum. In order to stimulate the prostate gland, press against the front wall of the rectum with a slight downward pressure. At the same time, apply firm pressure behind the scrotum with the heel of your hand.

STIMULATING A WOMAN

Using very gentle pressure, insert a well-lubricated finger into the rectum or move it gently in and out. Keep the heel of your hand pressed firmly between the anus and the vulva. As you apply pressure from the outside, ask your partner to bear down on your finger. This deliberate action may help to tighten up the anal sphincter and then allow it to relax.

Once you insert your finger into the rectum, keep it away from the vagina, and wash it thoroughly as soon as possible afterward.

SEXUAL AIDS

Men and women respond romantically and erotically to environment, ambience, and atmosphere. There is little question that soft lighting, subdued colors, gentle background music, pleasing scents, melodious voices, and soft and sexy clothes help reduce inhibitions and increase the possibility of intimacy. There are, however, a variety of other devices and techniques that add to sexual pleasure and, for some people, may be a necessity.

VIBRATORS

The first vibrators were based on the dildo, an artificial penis that has been used by both sexes for many thousands of years. The most recent variation on the traditional dildo is the battery-operated vibrator, which is sold widely in sex shops. Vibrators are used mostly to

MEN AND VIBRATORS

It is unlikely that a vibrator will have the explosive effect on a man that it has on a woman, though it can heighten pleasure enormously in sensitive spots.

The area just behind the root of the penis and in front of the anus is extremely sensitive to deep vibration, and a vibrator used there will increase sexual pleasure enormously. Almost all of the shaft of the penis, particularly the undersurface, is sensitive to vibration, too, and this rises as the tip is approached. Sensation is intense around the frenulum and so arousing when vibration is over the tip that it can be used as a cure for impotence (see Success With Sexual Problems).

WOMEN AND VIBRATORS

A woman who can't reach orgasm during intercourse often wonders if there is something physically wrong with her that prevents her from reaching orgasm. A self-induced orgasm answers that question in a few minutes, and it is here that a vibrator may be truly useful. There is certainly nothing wrong with, and virtually no difference between, an orgasm reached with a vibrator and one reached during sexual intercourse. More importantly, a self-induced orgasm provides the emotional and physical foundation for having orgasms during intercourse.

A vibrator, therefore, can tear down the barriers of guilt, shame, and prudery that prevent so many women from finding the sexual fulfillment that they deserve. Some women have for years subconsciously imposed the same kind of paralysis on their sex organs as on their minds. An electric vibrator provides intense, almost unbearable sexual excitement, sufficient to overwhelm emotional obstacles, and makes the brain and the genital organs respond explosively in unison.

stimulate a woman's clitoris, and they can be a big help in cases when a woman otherwise has difficulty reaching orgasm during sexual intercourse.

The vibrator works by stimulating the millions of sensory nerve endings in the skin of the woman's labia and the clitoris, and a man can apply it to his penis and surrounding area to heighten his sensations there, too.

During intercourse, the penis pushes and pulls against the labia and clitoris and, so to speak, flicks on millions of tiny switches which fire off electric impulses to the brain. In a basic sense, the more sensors the penis stimulates, the greater the sexual sensations. Sad though it may be, a vibrator is better than most penises; in a given moment it can trigger at least a million more sensors than the most educated penis, and that means orgasm is virtually inevitable. This does not mean that a vibrator is necessary, or that the penis is useless. The whole idea of self-produced orgasm is simply to pave the way for satisfying sexual intercourse.

CREAMS AND LUBRICANTS

The vagina produces a natural lubricating fluid within a few seconds of being effectively sexually stimulated. This normally makes penetration by the penis easier and pleasurable. However, if a man does not persist with foreplay long enough, the vagina won't be given the chance to produce lubrication. Some women, too, do not produce enough lubricant and most, at different times in their lives (for instance after childbirth and after menopause), will produce less secretions than usual. At these times, an artificial lubricant may be used, and creams and jellies that are water-soluble are widely sold.

Creams and lubricants come in handy, too, when anal stimulation or intercourse is contemplated, and when manually stimulating your partner. Many men use them during masturbation to ease friction and enhance pleasure. During massage, too, scented oils or creams can add to the sensations.

Many women feel pressured not just by society or their partners but also by their own feelings about the presence or absence of lubrication as a sign of arousal. It is comforting to remember that erection of the clitoris and lubrication of the vagina, even erection of the penis, are merely reflexes that do not always accurately reflect our emotional or aroused state. Women can be intensely aroused without being well lubricated, and men can be intensely aroused without an erection. A well-lubricated vagina, seen solely as an opening for an erect penis, is an untenable sexist viewpoint.

APHRODISIACS

An aphrodisiac is a drug or substance that increases sexual desire. Despite powerful folklore and considerable effort to find such a substance, no proven, reliable aphrodisiacal drug has ever been found, though a wide variety of chemical products, animal and plant extracts, and foods have their devotees. Such substances only leave a temporary impression of well-being, which may well be due to the person's faith in them. Spanish Fly or cantharides, if taken internally, causes excruciating irritation to the intestine and to the gastric-urinary tract, especially of the mucus membranes of the urethra. The resulting irritation can cause death in either sex.

Love potions made from bits of animals, narcotics, amulets in phallic form, and pornographic pictures all have been used in an attempt to artificially stimulate sexual desire. So far no universal aphrodisiac has been found, and, in view of the diversity and complexity of individual tastes, it is unlikely that there ever will be. Real aphrodisiacs are the subtle physical and emotional factors that will revive sexual desire when it is low, such as intense love fantasies, erotic dreams, or a particularly attractive quality in a partner.

EROTIC MATERIAL

Reading or watching sexually explicit material can produce genital sensations in both women and men, and can have an effect on sexual behavior. Many men use pornography as an aid to masturbation, and many women find that racy material increases their interest in having sex, though few will admit to it.

If you are open and talk to your partner about your reactions to erotic stimuli, you will discover that you have many areas in common, including those things that turn you both on or off. If we can free ourselves from the social mores of the past, the emphasis on the mechanical in early sex books, and our own engraved perspectives, we will find that we are always in a situation to be turned on. It is reassuring to realize that in any situation we can control our sexual response, through our own selection of stimuli, by sharing with our partners, and by being aware of the different needs we have for love. In realizing this we liberate ourselves.

If, however, you subject your partner to pressure to watch material she or he finds offensive, or you force your partner to join in sexual activities that she or he doesn't enjoy, then the problems involved go far beyond your sex life. What is at stake is more likely to be whether either of you wants to continue in a relationship in which one person's views and preferences are given unequal weight, and whether the other is willing to change his or her attitude.

FANTASIES

Everyone fantasizes: women, men, and children. It would be very odd if we didn't, because fantasy is a form of sexual rehearsal along paths that are familiar and also some that are entirely new and imaginary. We all respond to fantasies because the most important organ of sexual pleasure is the brain. The brain, as the seat of emotions, can be responsible for either turning us on or off sex. If we are full of resentment, grief-stricken, angry, anxious, or miserable, the most attractive person in the world will not seem so, and any amount of foreplay will not arouse us. On the other hand, being sexually aware,

MEN'S FANTASIES

- Being involved in group sex.
- Watching others having sex.
- Making love in public where others can see.
- Having sex with a woman other than one's usual partner; she can be a celebrity, neighbor, past lover, or friend.
- Watching two women you know making love together; one could be one's partner, the other a relative, friend, or neighbor.
- Being forced by a woman to have sex.
- Forcing a woman to have intercourse against her will.
- Forcing a woman to have oral sex against her will.
- Making love in an unusual place.
- Being part of a threesome with another man and a woman.
- Being part of a threesome with two women.
- Having a homosexual encounter.
- Watching one or more men having sex with other women.
- Being sexually abused by a woman.
- Making love to a virgin.
- Having sex with a woman with enormous breasts.
- Making love outdoors, on a famous monument, for instance.
- Having a woman urinate on oneself.
- Having a woman use a dildo on oneself in order to have anal sex.

WOMEN'S FANTASIES

- Making love with one's partner.
- Making love with a former lover or someone other than one's present partner.
- Having sex in an exotic location.
- Being made to have sex against one's will.
- Having sex in public while being watched by others.
- Taking part in group sex.
- Making love with a complete stranger.
- Having sex with a partner of a different race.
- Making love to another woman.
- Being taken from behind by a stranger and never seeing the man's face.
- Stripping in public.
- Sexual activities involving an animal, particularly a horse or dog.
- Watching others having sex.
- Watching your regular partner having sex with another woman, or another man.
- Having a male slave.
- Taking part in a threesome, either with another man or with another woman, and one's usual partner.
- Having sex in unusual circumstances, for example, in a courtroom.
- Working as a prostitute and having a large number of clients to satisfy.
- Being tied down and taken forcibly against one's will.

being interested in sex, thinking about it, and, more importantly, fantasizing about it all will be arousing. In this sense, it would seem that the brain is the most crucial sex organ because it can override our sexual urges in any direction, either by turning them off, or by turning them on. Fantasies, therefore, are one of the cheapest and most effective sexual aids.

The best sexual fantasies, the ones that offer maximum pleasure, center around ideal situations — ones that are, for practical purposes, unobtainable in "real" life. And, also unlike real life, they can be turned on and off at will, either to accelerate or dampen sexual activity. Often, we use fantasy to concentrate our minds on what is actually happening to us during our own lovemaking. We "see" what is happening as well as experiencing it. This helps to focus our attention on our own sexual responses, making them larger than life, and encourages the brain to respond even more enthusiastically to the signals of arousal it is receiving. It then sends out hormones that increase the excitement in our genital organs.

Many people don't fantasize in terms of stories but in terms of sexual images, and, while some people would have difficulty confessing their fantasies, others are quite willing to discuss a particular set of mental images.

In rare cases, a person can become so fixed on a particular fantasy that he or she cannot become aroused without it. While a fantasy that exercises such a strong hold can be very useful during masturbation, it can get in the way of shared sexual activities. Instead of concentrating on how your partner is reacting, and what you can do to please him or her, you can become fixed on bringing your fantasy to life, and thus seem remote and nonresponsive.

SHARING FANTASIES

Some people think anything that turns their partners on is fine, and therefore join in a fantasy once it has been recounted; others may find that they can never cope with the desires expressed, and this can put considerable pressure on the relationship. Men, particularly, may have problems accepting their partners' fantasies, because they feel they are providing the "real thing." If she has such a partner, a woman should proceed with caution since he could take her fantasy as a criticism of his lovemaking. Usually, however, a relationship can be improved by building fantasy behavior into lovemaking, even if it is in a diluted form. After all, part of the appeal of a fantasy is that it is a form of exceptional behavior, which neither the creator nor his or her partner may ever want interpreted realistically. Most people would not want to engage in the kind of behavior they fantasize about, particularly the more bizarre practices.

Sharing fantasies is another way of personalizing your relationship; using them, you can tailor sexual behavior to your own needs and create a unique experience. But while sharing fantasies can teach you a lot about what excites your partner, it also may be fraught with problems. The behavior projected in a fantasy often must be scaled down to be socially acceptable. For instance, when women have fantasies involving rape and bondage what they would like is some increased ardor from their partners, not sex with violence; and when men reveal fantasies in which women dominate them sexually, they want sympathy, not scorn, from their partners. Therefore, if you are in doubt about what to share, bide your time until you see the situation more clearly.

The brain is our most powerful sexual organ. It enables us to have sex any place, any time, and with our choice of sexual partner

Sharing fantasies
Shared fantasies can be introduced into a long-term sexual relationship to add new excitement and rekindle arousal.

Fantasies allow us to free up sexual patterns and engage in new activities

HOW MEN USE FANTASIES

Fantasies are a vital part of a man's lovemaking and from early on play an important role in his sexual behaviour. As an adolescent, a man requires a series of images for arousal during masturbation, and some are provided by pornographic magazines and videos, others through mental activity. Later on, when achieving and maintaining an erection becomes more difficult, fantasies may be important to revive flagging ardor. Or, if a man has trouble achieving an erection at all, he will often use fantasies of a particularly erotic nature to help solve the problem. Often, a man will have a favorite fantasy, one that will arouse him without fail and which, because it is so personal, he may be reluctant to reveal for fear of its losing its potency.

FANTASY WOMEN

Men's fantasies are more widely known than women's because they've been more openly expressed. The women men tend to fantasize about are more a creation of soft-porn publications than any woman they have known. The women of male fantasies are often young, sexually insatiable, readily available, unashamedly exposed, and very experienced sexually. If they were able to express any preferences, they would be delighted with whatever a man did to them, and they would be begging for more.

In addition to the ever-available woman, probably the most common fantasy among men is the presence of more than one partner at the same time, exciting his body in different ways. So-called "perverse" fantasies are also common, especially after middle age, and deviant behavior such as homosexuality, transvestism, transsexuality, or pedophilia may be the theme. Bondage and anal sex are also imagined, and often this is a sign of obvious aggression toward one's partner.

HOW WOMEN USE FANTASIES

Fantasies give women butterflies in the stomach, make their skin tingle and their vaginas moisten. Women who prepare themselves for sexual encounters by thinking occasionally of the evening ahead while making their preparations — bathing, grooming, choosing clothes, using scent — are more easily aroused and enjoy sex more than women who do not make such preparations.

Just as men do, women use fantasies while masturbating and also to fuel flagging ardor. One-half of all women fantasize when making love, and only a few less than that do so regularly and frequently. Women who rate themselves as good lovers are more likely to use fantasy than those who rate themselves as poor lovers, and this makes sense in that fantasy is a valuable and powerful weapon against sexual repression. Many women find that it helps them to reach orgasm on occasions when they wouldn't otherwise.

MEN WOMEN FANTASIZE ABOUT

Women most often fantasize about another man known to them or imaginary lovers. This type of fantasy allows a woman to introduce variety into her sex life without undue effort or threatening an existing relationship. Such a lover is normally idealized and free of her partner's inadequacies or deficiencies.

Fantasies about a dream lover are followed closely by making love in some exotic location; a sun-drenched beach seems to be the favorite. Fantasies such as these can be seen as relief from the more boring aspects of normal day-to-day living.

Just as men do, women fantasize about being involved with more than one lover, and also about being forced to perform various "wicked" or "forbidden" acts. Fantasizing about being forced to have sex is a way of dealing with any subconscious guilt feelings that may be present as a result of poor sex education.

The Experience Of Making Love

BEING A GOOD LOVER

While a large part of being a good lover is to make and keep a relationship exciting, which depends on exploring and mastering a range of sexual activities, to my mind, the primary task is to satisfy each other's emotional needs. I am convinced that real sexual happiness is not the direct result of technical ability but depends on you having positive feelings about your own sexuality and that of your partner. The best sex happens in the best relationships. True sexual chemistry can develop only when partners are attracted to each other as individuals, not just as representatives of the opposite sex. With affection, honesty, and trust, partners should explore and develop their sexuality together, bearing in mind the likes and dislikes they each have.

A man often forgets that a woman is both sentimental and sensual, so that her idea of lovemaking includes a prologue of emotions tenderly exchanged. In order to recapture these feelings, it helps to look back to the time when you first fell in love, when just sitting together talking or in companionable silence was enough. I'm sure you will agree there was pleasure in every treasured sign of affection — touches, looks, nuzzles, gentle caresses, and kisses. You will have greater pleasure and satisfaction if you remember these earlier emotions when the time comes to arouse another intensely.

—— COMMUNICATION IS IMPORTANT ——

No one can know instinctively what his or her partner enjoys. It is up to each of us to talk about our likes and dislikes; it is not unnecessary, and it is not insulting. It is almost impossible to have a good sexual relationship without clear communication.

We should all let our partners know which caresses are pleasurable, and which are not. We should always say if something is very arousing or painful. Lovers should be bold enough to suggest a different way of making love, and ask each other questions and make requests. Exchanging these confidences helps to build a better physical relationship, while not doing so may make matters irrevocably worse. This can be achieved by saying that something is pleasant or it is not, making encouraging noises, or by moving a hand to a spot where the sensation is more pleasurable.

What is appropriate and enjoyable varies from occasion to occasion, so simply because you have expressed a preference once does not mean to say that you do not have to express it again, or that you might express a different preference on a different occasion. Good lovers should never take each other for granted.

Ideally, when conflicting desires are expressed, or when differing degrees of arousal are experienced, a couple should engage in a process of negotiation. If not, you will find yourselves falling into habitual, routine sexual activities. The best of partners may eventually become bored after years of exactly the same activity in the same sequence, in the same position, in the same bed. Boring sex is rarely rewarding to either partner, and there is a considerable range of sexual activities that people find appealing and stimulating.

Communication does not mean that everything said has to be negative. The best kind of communication is to say what pleases you and at the same time, to listen to what your partner is telling you.

And if you want to get more enjoyment out of your sexual relationship, you need a partner's full involvement and participation. For two people to fully enjoy their sexual relationship both must be able to accept the pleasure a partner gives, and both must be able to enjoy the process of giving a partner pleasure. The most satisfying sexual relationships have the joint commitment of the two people involved. The more pleasure you receive from your partner the more they will want to give pleasure in return. A good sexual relationship is always a giving relationship, not a taking one.

— TALKING OPENLY ABOUT DESIRES —

An amazing number of people find it difficult to talk directly and honestly with their partners about their sexual desires, fears, and problems. Many people have been trained to perceive discussions about sex as being so private, so embarrassing, and so revealing that they hesitate to talk about their own feelings and wishes even with the person they've been married to for years.

In this context it is absolutely essential for partners to talk to each other about sex, so that their bodies can adjust mutually and their pleasures increase. Despite this, in my experience, most couples never talk to each other about what they do in bed, whether it is good or bad, or whether it gives them any satisfaction. I, for one, find it hard to believe that during the most intense moments of a couple's relationship, neither partner knows what the other is thinking; their minds remain separate whereas their bodies are striving to get as close as two bodies can.

Many women talk freely to their friends about unfulfilled desires, disappointments, and frustrations, but men generally keep their sex lives secret. I'm certain there would be far fewer misunderstandings, arguments, and conflicts if both partners would talk openly about their physical and emotional expectations. I believe that nothing but good would come of sharing these innermost desires, however strange and fantastic they might appear to be.

MEN AS LOVERS

Many men, no matter what else they may be, are not skillful lovers. Research has shown time and again that the most consistent complaint made by women is that their partners do not take enough time for foreplay. Most sexual relationships are built on mutual trust and respect, and have been developing on a friendly basis for some time. Most couples have shared a gradually deepening physical intimacy stopping at petting. During this time, both partners are anxious to please each other. They find that they communicate exceptionally well because messages are important, and they need to be explained and understood. This gradual exploration and development of understanding means that couples are sexually relaxed the first time they try intercourse. But over time, with many men seeing penetration as the goal to be reached as quickly as possible, talking and foreplay dwindle, to the universal disappointment of women.

MEETING WOMEN'S NEEDS

What the majority of men don't seem to understand is that during foreplay the progress from kissing and cuddling to caressing the breasts, nipples, and clitoris is not only very exciting and pleasurable for a woman, and incidentally to most men, it is absolutely necessary for a woman's arousal, and always crucial to her sexual pleasure and satisfaction. Without it, a woman is not sexually aroused, is not an uninhibited participant, is not even physiologically ready in terms of lubrication. But worse, after intercourse she remains unsatisfied, resentful, and wide awake while her partner turns over and goes to sleep. In a way, men and women are mismatched in this respect because a man is much more easily and quickly aroused, and reaches orgasm in an extremely short time under almost any circumstances. Is it any wonder that sex can end up being a battleground, often a silent one, and becomes more and more uninteresting and infrequent? A couple can become embarrassingly out of step, and sex becomes something to be missed rather than looked forward to and sought after.

PERFECTING YOUR TECHNIQUE

Some of the things women say about men indicate what they would like to see changed.

"I'd like him to touch me all over a lot more — more foreplay, more heavy petting, more kissing everywhere, and more oral sex";

"I love my breasts and nipples to be fondled and caressed, and I always wondered if I could have a climax just by being played with, but my partner is too impatient";

"My partner thinks kissing isn't manly."

Men should be sensual as well as sexual and many find it hard to spend time on purely pleasurable activities and feel uneasy about engaging in enjoyable experiences. To overcome this, when giving caresses, think of the pleasure you are providing to a loved one. Most women find foreplay hugely enjoyable, and see hugs and kisses as the true signs of affection. Try to discover your partner's most sensitive areas and the kind of stimulation she prefers — gentle or slightly rougher.

Don't be afraid to relax and let your partner take the initiative. Let her know, in words or gestures, what feels particularly good and, if necessary, guide her hand with yours. Try to concentrate on what you feel and the proximity of her body as she touches you. Respond to your feelings by moving, breathing more heavily, or expressing pleasure verbally. Most women find a responsive man very exciting. Don't always feel that you have to be successful at every sexual encounter; you will just find the occasional failure too hard to take. Most women are understanding about an occasional failure, and even view it as an opportunity to show their love.

WOMEN AS LOVERS

While we know that men are easily aroused and reach orgasm more quickly and easily than women, not all are as sexually straightforward as many women believe.

MEETING MEN'S NEEDS

I have no doubt that men also need the excitement and gratification derived from an emotional involvement in lovemaking. There is hardly a man who does not need to feel loved, admired, and physically cherished if he is to experience the true depths of sexual pleasure with his partner. Yet far too many women place the entire responsibility of initiating and orchestrating sex on men. Traditionally, the man suggests sex and the woman either accepts or rejects him, and in this way the man usually determines how much sex a couple has. This amounts to a great deal of pressure, and many sensitive men do not really relish having such a heavy burden. Better sex and happier couples ensue when partners feel equally free to suggest or refuse sex, and do so equally often. If you take the initiative in suggesting sex and expect to be both accepted and refused, you are much less likely to feel guilty on occasions when your partner wants to have sex and you don't, and less likely to feel angry and rejected when you want to have sex and he doesn't.

Taking responsibility for suggesting sex also means that lovemaking will result more from inclination rather than obligation. Women easily can say "yes" to sex but remain uninvolved. For a man, a compliant but unresponsive woman will never be as sensual, exciting, or as satisfying as a woman who is involved and skillful.

PERFECTING YOUR TECHNIQUE

To be a good sexual partner means that you should keep sex vital and interesting, not only by regarding it as the best means of expressing your affection toward your partner, but also by experimenting with a variety of techniques and practices. You always should be willing to take the initiative. Don't always leave the first move to your partner. Men want to feel that they are accepted by their partners, and worth some effort to arouse and delight. Try some seduction occasionally; tell your partner to lie back and enjoy your caresses as you take the active part.

Remember always to communicate your enjoyment of what you are doing or what is being done to you. Don't be embarrassed about the way you look and sound while making love. Almost all men find expressions of desire and signs of growing sexual excitement in women very stimulating. A lot of women give too little feedback to their partners so that men feel discouraged and unappreciated for what they are doing and will, in future, pay less attention to foreplay.

Use your imagination as much as possible. This is especially important in long-term relationships when boredom can easily wear away at sexual enjoyment. In addition to picking and choosing among the entire range of the normal sexual repertoire (see page 55), introduce activities that will bring some novelty into your relationship. Try suggesting taking a bath or shower together; make love outdoors in a private place; plan lunch at home but make love instead; abandon your bed in favor of the floor, sofa, or a rug; use a mirror to watch yourselves making love, or view a sexy video together; or devote time to a sexual banquet of both partners' choosing.

Show enthusiasm toward your partner's suggestions for enlivening your sex life. Most human sexual activity is reassuringly ordinary, and unless something is painful or distressing, it is worth finding out whether it gives you pleasure. In sex, as in all things, let your instincts be your guide.

VARYING EXPERIENCES

Earlier we looked at the individual experiences of men and women in achieving orgasm. But, as with all the best love play, orgasms should be a shared experience. That doesn't mean, however, they must occur necessarily at the same time.

Some couples feel erroneously that only a simultaneous orgasm is the perfect one. This is a romantic notion that doesn't work for all lovers. At climax, you move to a different level of consciousness, and you become totally absorbed in the experience. If you are prevented from doing so because you need to know where your partner is, you may not be able to manage a climax at all, or you may have a less satisfying one. And, for many lovers, watching the other experiencing his or her orgasm is the greatest of sexual turn-ons.

For most couples, the attainment of simultaneous orgasms only happens now and then, and sex is no less enjoyable for that. Seeking simultaneous orgasms should not become obsessive. There are many patterns of successful lovemaking which exclude simultaneous orgasms (and some that exclude all orgasms), but nonetheless draw couples very close and have infinite positive effects on everyday experiences as well as on social and family life.

And then there are the exceptional circumstances — prolonged and multiple orgasms — that are quite rare unless both partners are aware of each other's sexual needs and are generous enough to look after them. Most couples find these forms of sexual intercourse the most exciting and sexually satisfying, but they take quite a bit of practice and are most often found within long-term relationships. Partners must be very familiar with each other and have planned and worked to reach a state of sexual sophistication.

PROLONGED ORGASM

This can be practiced only if a man is able to control his ejaculatory reflex at will. It is a form of sexual union usually indulged in by partners who have been making love together for some time, know each other well, and have learned how to adjust to each other's needs. This can be one of the most exciting forms of sexual union, and is one of the most treasured aspects of a long-term loving relationship.

For it to occur, the woman must be highly aroused during foreplay and then the sexual tension of both partners must be maintained by intermittent thrusting movements, punctuated by pauses from time to time for as long as each partner wishes. When sensation reaches a peak and can't be put off further, both partners enjoy orgasm in a mutually agreed-upon, final burst of lovemaking.

MULTIPLE ORGASMS

Until recently, we believed that only women were capable of multiple orgasms, but new research has shown that some men are able to have them, too. Since orgasm is not necessarily synonymous with ejaculation, but is more accurately defined as the intense and diffuse pleasurable sensations the man feels, it is perfectly possible for a man to have several climaxes in fairly quick succession. For a man's experience of multiple orgasm to be similar to a woman's, he should have two or more orgasms, with or without ejaculation, and with only very limited, if any, detumescence.

THE MAN'S EXPERIENCE

Doctors have documented the experiences of multiorgasmic men who had from two to nine orgasms per session. Some ejaculated at the first orgasm, some at the last, and the rest in between; some even ejaculated more than once. Many of the men first experienced multiple orgasms in middle age.

Probably, more men could become multiorgasmic if they overcome the conditioning that says they will only ejaculate and then detumesce. A nondemanding atmosphere, emotional closeness, and the opportunity for leisurely sex will improve a man's chances of experiencing multiple orgasms, as will having a partner who is sexually responsive and does not tire of prolonged intercourse.

However, just as with multiorgasmic women, men who are capable of more than one orgasm will not be able to or want to experience them at every sexual encounter.

A man can practice becoming multiorgasmic by coming to the brink of orgasm yet inhibiting ejaculation until he can separate the two sensations. In the relaxed atmosphere of a loving relationship, some men will find that they don't necessarily lose their erections, and they will be able to achieve additional climaxes. However, few men have the desire to gain such training in self-control, or appreciate dry orgasms, because for most men climax involves ejaculation.

THE WOMAN'S EXPERIENCE

For a woman to enjoy multiple orgasms, her man must exercise careful control to avoid ejaculating, yet provide her with deep and rapid thrusting sufficient for her to achieve orgasm. Or, a woman may use a vibrator, or she or her partner may masturbate her. After each orgasm, both partners rest a while and then the cycle can begin again until she signals that she is ready for him to climax inside her. In this way, a woman can enjoy two, three, or many more orgasms. In the best of all possible worlds, her partner will climax simultaneously with her last one, though often the rigid control needed means that he experiences his own orgasm only when his partner is fully satisfied.

Most women find that they can build up their level of sexual arousal with practice; the more a woman masturbates, the more pleasure she gets from it, and the more she will want to do so. Most women can improve their potentials for multiple orgasm by keeping their pelvic muscles in good condition, and sharing fantasies, but, above all, they need to encourage their partners to help them. If you are trying to have multiple orgasms, your partner needs to know, and you should encourage him to continue stimulating you in the way you like best, even after you've had an initial climax. Because a man's experience of orgasm is so different, your partner may think you have had enough of love play just because he has.

SYNCHRONIZING ORGASMS

THE MAN'S EXPERIENCE Although he has always enjoyed having sex with his partner, this man feels that he has matured greatly in his attitude over the years. Although when he was younger he believed that sex was mainly for male pleasure, he has discovered, with the help of his partner, that sex is infinitely better if both partners actively enjoy each other's bodies. He loves being able to give his partner pleasure, and he is happy that she is so responsive to him. And while he often has to lose touch with his own feelings in concentrating so hard upon his partner's pleasures that he can't relax and enjoy his own orgasm as much as he'd like, he doesn't want to become selfish, so he tries to achieve the occasional simultaneous orgasm.

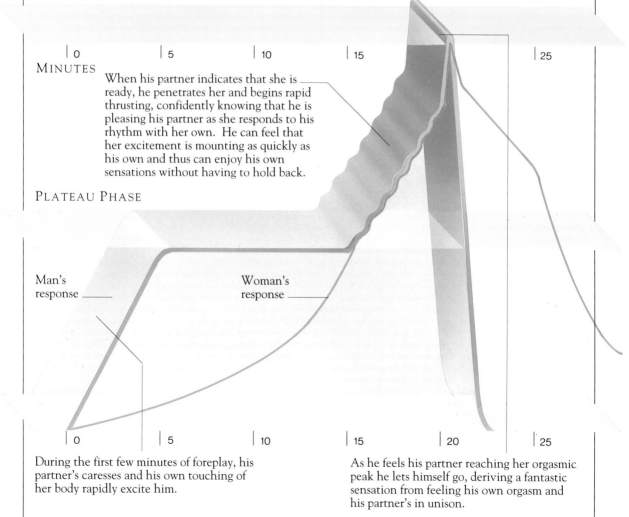

ORGASM

MINUTES | 0   5   10   15   25

When his partner indicates that she is ready, he penetrates her and begins rapid thrusting, confidently knowing that he is pleasing his partner as she responds to his rhythm with her own. He can feel that her excitement is mounting as quickly as his own and thus can enjoy his own sensations without having to hold back.

PLATEAU PHASE

Man's response ———

Woman's response ———

0   5   10   15   20   25

During the first few minutes of foreplay, his partner's caresses and his own touching of her body rapidly excite him.

As he feels his partner reaching her orgasmic peak he lets himself go, deriving a fantastic sensation from feeling his own orgasm and his partner's in unison.

THE WOMAN'S EXPERIENCE This woman initially never could relax enough
to really enjoy sex with her partner. Over the years, however, she has discovered that
sex can fulfill the romantic ideal which she had always held. Learning through
gentle exploration and the sharing of ideas with her partner, she has become aware of
the sensations that stimulate her own body. Relaxed, confident, and uninhibited,
she can communicate her wishes to her partner through touches which excite them
both and ensure that their excitement meets. Though she doesn't feel it is necessary
to be obsessive about achieving orgasm together, every once in a while, as here, she is
able to achieve simultaneous orgasm with her partner.

ORGASM

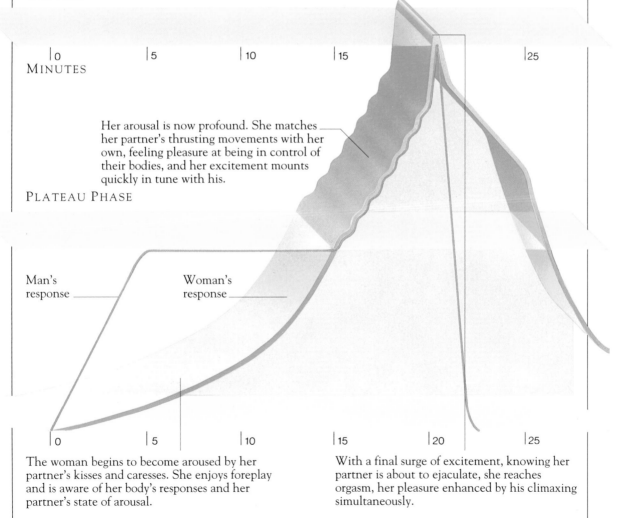

MINUTES
| 0 | 5 | 10 | 15 | 25 |

Her arousal is now profound. She matches
her partner's thrusting movements with her
own, feeling pleasure at being in control of
their bodies, and her excitement mounts
quickly in tune with his.

PLATEAU PHASE

Man's
response

Woman's
response

| 0 | 5 | 10 | 15 | 20 | 25 |

The woman begins to become aroused by her
partner's kisses and caresses. She enjoys foreplay
and is aware of her body's responses and her
partner's state of arousal.

With a final surge of excitement, knowing her
partner is about to ejaculate, she reaches
orgasm, her pleasure enhanced by his climaxing
simultaneously.

PROLONGED ORGASM

THE MAN'S EXPERIENCE   This man has been making love to his partner for a number of years. In the early stages of their relationship, he was very involved with his job and regarded sex as a way to work off some of his frustrations and tension. It was only when he began to succeed at work that he began to pay more attention to whether his partner was finding sex as satisfying as he did. He found he could increase the pleasure they both felt substantially by controlling his orgasm and maintaining sexual tension for as long as possible.

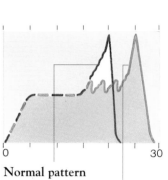

Normal pattern

Prolonged orgasm

ORGASM

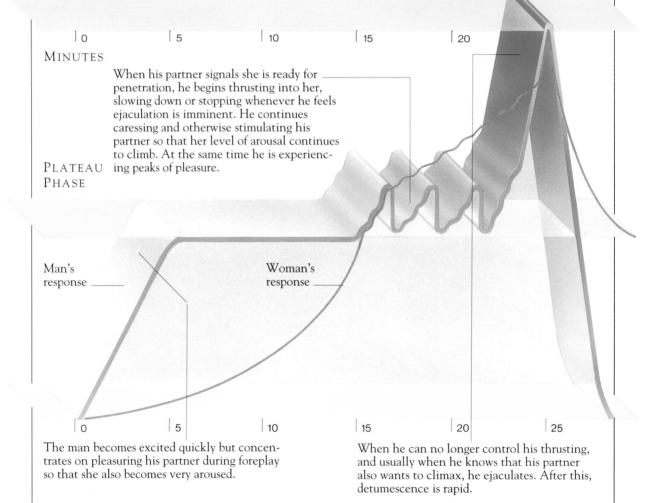

MINUTES

When his partner signals she is ready for penetration, he begins thrusting into her, slowing down or stopping whenever he feels ejaculation is imminent. He continues caressing and otherwise stimulating his partner so that her level of arousal continues to climb. At the same time he is experiencing peaks of pleasure.

PLATEAU
PHASE

Man's
response

Woman's
response

The man becomes excited quickly but concentrates on pleasuring his partner during foreplay so that she also becomes very aroused.

When he can no longer control his thrusting, and usually when he knows that his partner also wants to climax, he ejaculates. After this, detumescence is rapid.

THE WOMAN'S EXPERIENCE

This woman often wished that intercourse could last longer, and in a relationship with a partner to whom she had been making love for several years, this became possible. Both partners became attuned to each other's bodies and could read each other's signals as to what was wanted. The woman encouraged her partner to thrust into her without ejaculating and having an orgasm until she felt satiated, and in this way they were able to have prolonged, mutually satisfying, and stimulating sex.

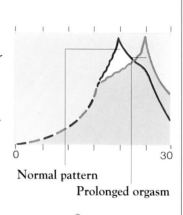

0   30

Normal pattern

Prolonged orgasm

ORGASM

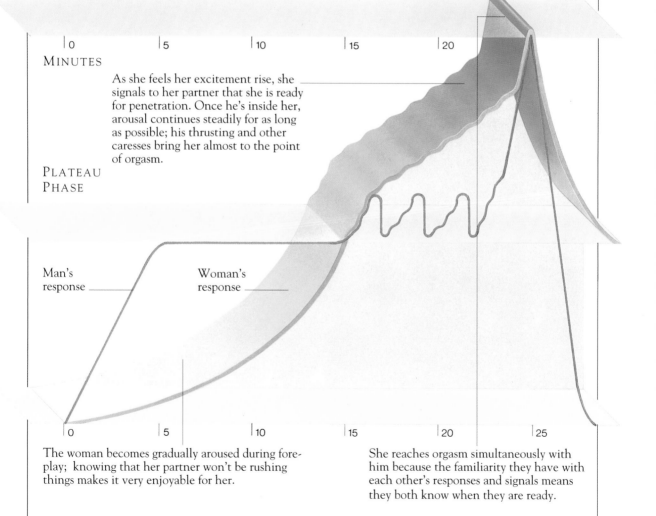

| 0 | 5 | 10 | 15 | 20

MINUTES

As she feels her excitement rise, she signals to her partner that she is ready for penetration. Once he's inside her, arousal continues steadily for as long as possible; his thrusting and other caresses bring her almost to the point of orgasm.

PLATEAU
PHASE

Man's response ——

Woman's response ——

| 0 | 5 | 10 | 15 | 20 | 25

The woman becomes gradually aroused during foreplay; knowing that her partner won't be rushing things makes it very enjoyable for her.

She reaches orgasm simultaneously with him because the familiarity they have with each other's responses and signals means they both know when they are ready.

MULTIPLE ORGASMS

THE MAN'S EXPERIENCE This man enjoys a good sex life with his partner, and has always felt that pleasing her could only add to his own pleasure. In his mature years, he has become more open about discussing what she would like, and more able to control his own sexual excitement. Whether or not his ejaculatory control is due to the aging process, he has been pleased to discover that by holding back on his ejaculation, he can achieve peaks of pleasure before his final climax, and can induce multiple orgasms and, therefore, great sexual fulfillment in his partner.

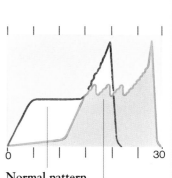

Normal pattern

Multiple orgasms

ORGASM

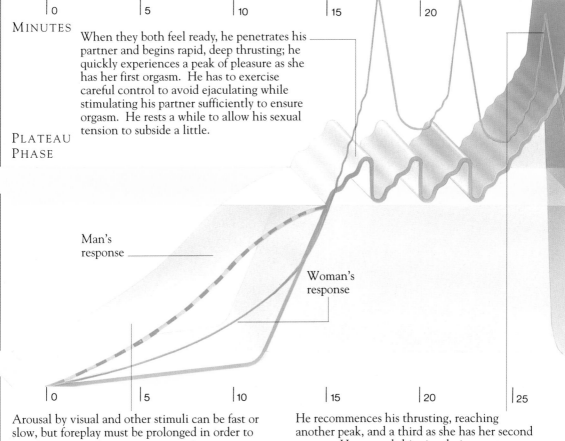

MINUTES

PLATEAU
PHASE

When they both feel ready, he penetrates his partner and begins rapid, deep thrusting; he quickly experiences a peak of pleasure as she has her first orgasm. He has to exercise careful control to avoid ejaculating while stimulating his partner sufficiently to ensure orgasm. He rests a while to allow his sexual tension to subside a little.

Man's
response

Woman's
response

Arousal by visual and other stimuli can be fast or slow, but foreplay must be prolonged in order to give his partner the necessary stimulation.

He recommences his thrusting, reaching another peak, and a third as she has her second orgasm. He controls his ejaculation, rests again, and when ready, climaxes as his partner experiences her last orgasm.

THE WOMAN'S EXPERIENCE   This woman and her partner have built up a great intimacy and knowledge of each other's bodies, sexual desires, and needs. They have always communicated well with each other and found that as time goes by they have become less inhibited and have enjoyed a resurgence in sexual desire for each other. She used to think that multiple orgasms were myths, but as her partner has become a more careful and studied lover, and can control his own orgasm longer, she now frequently enjoys two or even three orgasms.

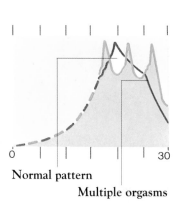

Normal pattern

Multiple orgasms

ORGASM

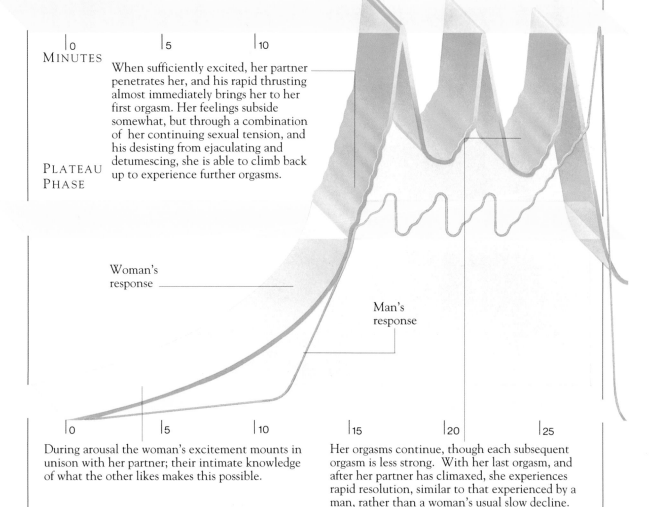

MINUTES

PLATEAU
PHASE

When sufficiently excited, her partner penetrates her, and his rapid thrusting almost immediately brings her to her first orgasm. Her feelings subside somewhat, but through a combination of her continuing sexual tension, and his desisting from ejaculating and detumescing, she is able to climb back up to experience further orgasms.

Woman's
response

Man's
response

During arousal the woman's excitement mounts in unison with her partner; their intimate knowledge of what the other likes makes this possible.

Her orgasms continue, though each subsequent orgasm is less strong. With her last orgasm, and after her partner has climaxed, she experiences rapid resolution, similar to that experienced by a man, rather than a woman's usual slow decline.

POSITIONS FOR MAKING LOVE

Often, when couples whose sex life has lost its sparkle consult me about making improvements, one of the first questions I ask is whether they vary the way they make love. Many of these couples have tied themselves to a single position for lovemaking, and it has become boring. The missionary position, with the man on top and the woman underneath, is most commonly used and, for some couples, never varied. It is so named because it was forcibly advocated by missionaries who took their faith to "heathen" or "uncivilized" peoples. For many years the church tolerated this position only, since it was thought to be the one in which the woman was almost certain to be fertilized. The position also allowed the man always to adopt the dominant role, and experience most or all of the pleasure.

But between consenting lovers, all coital positions are perfectly normal and legitimate, and the sex lives of us all will certainly be enlivened by a little adventure and experimentation.

CHOOSING A POSITION

There is no such thing as the best position; each couple should experiment and find their own most favorable positions, which will depend on the shape and size of the couple's bodies, both partners' strength and stamina, and any special situations such as a pregnancy, disability, or illness (see Loving Sex Throughout Life, page 150). Couples who are making love for the first time very often experiment with a variety of positions in quick succession in an attempt to satisfy their curiosity.

At the same time, partners should try to find out as much as they can about each other's body so that they can adjust to each other physically. One of the purposes that a book like this serves is to enlighten couples who are ignorant or lacking in imagination, and who cannot believe that there are other positions besides those they happen to have come across by chance. Remember that expertise cannot be attained in a day; it may take months of enjoyable experimentation before a couple finds the several positions which, for them, are wholly satisfying and fulfilling in every sense.

On the following pages are illustrated a great many positions that have benefits for one or both partners, and for a variety of reasons. Listed below, in no particular order, are some of the considerations that each partner in a couple looks for, and that the chosen positions must take into account.

Both partners should note the preferences of the other, which means that each has the responsibility for expressing his or her predilections in the first place. To enjoy intercourse to the maximum, however, any position in which it is tried should be comfortable and allow freedom of movement, and must accommodate the abilities of the less athletic partner.

Certain positions are uncomfortable or even painful for one partner, while others can increase the feeling of pleasure and enhance sexual arousal so that the chances of an orgasm for both partners, but especially the woman, are increased. This is not to say that any one particular position is better than another; each position may have its own advantages in any given situation, taking into account how each partner feels physically and emotionally.

THE MAN'S CHOICE OF POSITION

- Does it allow good penetration (shallow or deep, as desired)?
- Will he be able to see his partner's vulva?
- Will he have good access to his partner's clitoris?
- Can he reach her breasts with his hands or mouth?
- Can he move easily?
- Will it prolong intercourse or, if desired, is it good for a quick getaway?
- Is it tiring?
- Can his partner move?
- Does it allow for his unusually small or large penis?
- If he has erection difficulties, can the position be achieved without a firm erection?
- Can he kiss and cuddle his partner?
- Is it good if his partner is much heavier or lighter than himself?
- Does it need a lot of undressing?
- Does it allow him to take the dominant (or passive) role?
- Can he stimulate his partner's anal area ?
- Is it possible during pregnancy?

THE WOMAN'S CHOICE OF POSITION

- Can she move so that stimulation remains good?
- Does it allow her to see her partner?
- Is it comfortable during the latter stages of pregnancy?
- Can she or her partner reach her clitoris easily?
- Does it allow her to kiss her partner?
- Will it stimulate her G spot?
- Is it comfortable?
- Does it allow her partner to reach her breasts?
- In it, can she reach down and touch her partner's scrotum?
- Is it good for cuddling?
- Does it allow good skin contact?
- Is it good for conception?
- What sort of penetration does it allow, and does she want—shallow or deep?
- Is it good for learning sex with a new partner?
- Does it stimulate the back or front vaginal wall?
- Does it allow her to take a dominant (or submissive) role?
- Can she see and speak to her partner?

MAN-ON-TOP POSITIONS 1

Man-on-top positions, in particular the missionary position, where the man lies between the woman's thighs, are probably the most widely used of all sexual positions. They give the man almost total control over intercourse, but the woman is allowed very little freedom of movement.

Man-on-top positions are especially good for couples who are just beginning to have sex with each other, as there is full eye contact and the ability to communicate with each other so that preferences and responses can be noted. The other advantages they offer are plenty of scope for kissing, deep penetration, and manual stimulation, plus access to the male posterior. They are good also if conception is desirable.

She can use her leg to apply pressure to his back and buttocks, and for some control over his thrusting

1 Once he is erect, the man enters his partner directly so that his penis is parallel to her vaginal walls. If she spreads her legs wide, the stretchy feeling is quite sensuous.

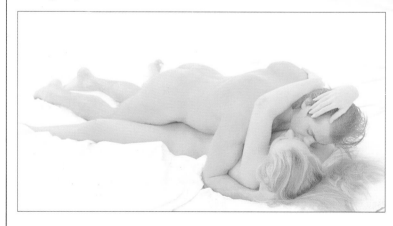

Face-to-face, the couple has full eye contact and can kiss passionately while they make love

He can take his weight on his elbows, allowing his partner to move her pelvis more freely

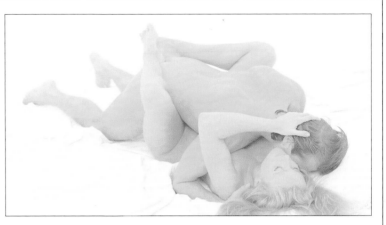

2 If the woman brings her leg up to apply pressure to her partner's back, she can control the depth and angle of his thrust, perhaps so that he presses on the front wall of her vagina, the site of her G spot.

3 By bringing up both legs to wrap them around her partner, a fit and supple woman alters the tilt of her pelvis, which can produce new sensations for both her and her partner, and increases genital contact.

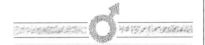

FOR THE MAN

Being on top has obvious advantages. He has wide access to his partner for kissing and caressing her upper body and breasts and, at the same time, the superior position allows him to control his thrusting, speeding up or slowing down as necessary.

FOR THE WOMAN

Man-on-top positions feed a woman's romantic needs. Here, she is obviously being made love to, and can lie back and enjoy the sensations. Being face-to-face positions, they are good for kissing, intimate talking, and caresses of all kinds.

MAN-ON-TOP POSITIONS 2

Man-on-top positions feed a man's need to dominate by allowing him to penetrate his partner deeply, and a woman's desire to be dominated because in them she takes the passive role. Most men enjoy penetrating a woman's body as deeply as possible, and women like it, too, especially when they are particularly aroused and want to be "filled up." And, when a woman opens herself completely to her partner, it makes him feel especially wanted. In these positions, the man can move freely to control the intensity and depth of his thrusts; the woman can add to his sensations by contracting and relaxing her muscles to "milk" her partner's penis.

1 As a variation from entering his partner from above, the man can kneel and approach her from a vertical position. He can thus push off against the bed into his partner. She helps increase contact by wrapping her legs around him tightly.

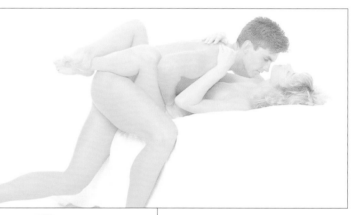

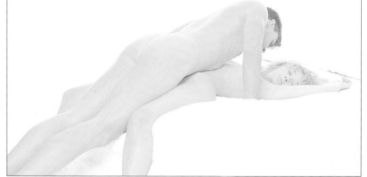

2 By sliding his partner down the side of the bed, the man can lean forward on her body, taking most of his weight on his forearms while she relaxes and lets herself be taken completely. Movement and penetration are limited so that arousal can be controlled.

FOR THE MAN

Using these positions the man is able to control his thrusting, and thus the speed at which he reaches orgasm. This kind of control is especially beneficial if the man is at all worried about losing his erection, or if he wants to delay ejaculation.

3 Finally, pushing them both up the bed, his knees thrusting her legs wide apart, the man can penetrate his partner quite deeply. For her, the sensation is increased by having her knees close to her chest and her bottom raised by a pillow.

FOR THE WOMAN

Being on her back is relaxing and allows the woman freedom to lie back and enjoy the sensations of being overpowered by her partner. It also "absolves" her from having to be responsible for what happens during sexual intercourse.

Deeply entwined, she feels secure enough to open herself completely to her partner

He uses his thigh and knee to give added pressure to the tempo and depth of his thrusts

When highly aroused, spreading her legs widely will make deep penetration easier

MAN-ON-TOP POSITIONS 3

Some of the more advanced man-on-top positions require a certain degree of suppleness and athleticism, and an accommodating partner. The most deeply penetrating positions are those where the woman's legs are against her chest; these should be avoided in the late stages of pregnancy. The positions below require the penis to be inserted at varying angles, which should produce new and different sensations.

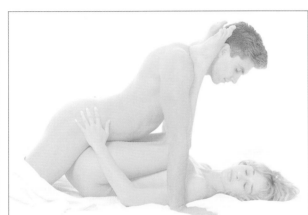

Woman's legs to chest position
She pulls her knees close to her chest and puts her feet on her partner's shoulders. With his weight on his hands, the man can push forward and penetrate his partner to the maximum amount while stimulating the back wall of her vagina.

Man sitting forward
He sits up with his legs widely spread and eases his partner onto his penis. The different sensations the man experiences by manipulating his partner up and down more than make up for the limited thrusting he can achieve here.

FOR THE MAN
Varying the angle of approach to his partner provides the man with satisfying and stimulating sensations. The less the woman is able to move, the more the man can control his level of excitement. Here he is in total control of the pace of intercourse.

FOR THE WOMAN
Variations on man-on-top positions provide variety while still permitting the woman to remain the passive party, if she so wishes. The deep penetration positions are good for conception but must be avoided in the late stages of pregnancy.

Face-to-face,
the couple can
communicate
their desires

The unusual
body angle
produces new
and different
sensations

She can caress
her partner's
body and enjoy
the sensations of
her partner's
penis pressing on
the side of her
vagina

Cross buttock position
Here it is the woman's turn to
experience some unusual sensations as her partner's penis
presses onto the side of her
vagina. The man can stay in this
position or rotate slowly toward
or away from his partner. This
position makes it easy to exchange information about which
movements are most pleasing.

WOMAN-ON-TOP POSITIONS 1

Both men and women find the woman-on-top positions extremely satisfying. They enable a woman to take a more active role in controlling both the sensations she gives and those she receives. With the man underneath and relatively immobile, she can stimulate his penis easily by moving up and down, and more readily control the depth of penetration. For the man, such positions prove that his partner is taking the lead; with them, he can feel himself the object of her active seduction.

Woman-on-top positions are also comfortable ones, particularly when the woman is much lighter than her partner.

He is the passive partner, feeling wanted and seduced, and can concentrate on his own arousal knowing that his partner is controlling her own stimulation

1 To get into the simplest position, where the woman lies on top of her partner with her legs outside, it is probably best to start from a side-by-side embrace. Then she needs to gently throw a leg across her partner's thighs and climb on top. The woman helps to guide her partner's penis inside her.

His hands can caress her back and buttocks, occasionally holding her to guide the angle of penetration

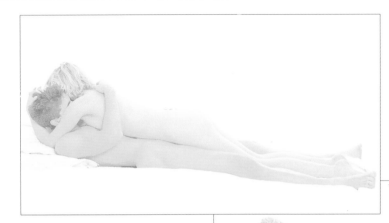

2 If the woman now brings her legs inside her partner's, this results in a snugger fit between both genital areas. If she keeps her legs tightly closed, she heightens the friction between the vagina and pelvis. She can add to the sensation by contracting her pelvic muscles.

3 Finally, if the woman spreads her legs out widely to the side, the pubic regions are perfectly aligned. From here, she can press down on her partner's feet, which is highly arousing to him because she is obviously "using" her partner in order to satisfy herself.

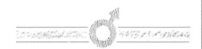

FOR THE MAN

He can lie back and enjoy sensations she arouses in him. This is particularly important where he can't take the lead sexually due to tiredness or illness.

She takes the active role, raising and lowering herself onto his erection

She can push his legs apart or together with hers, thus changing the sensations for both of them

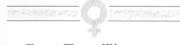

FOR THE WOMAN

As well as being ideal for a woman to please herself as she likes, these positions are useful when a partner is particularly large, or when she is pregnant.

WOMAN-ON-TOP POSITIONS 2

Woman-on-top positions in which the woman is sitting up have several advantages for both partners. The woman has full view of the man, and by taking all her weight on herself, she can more actively caress him while adjusting his penile movements to her liking. For the man, he is free to fondle his partner's freely moving breasts, which are held tantalizingly close to him, and he can see his penis entering her vagina; both sights are very exciting to him.

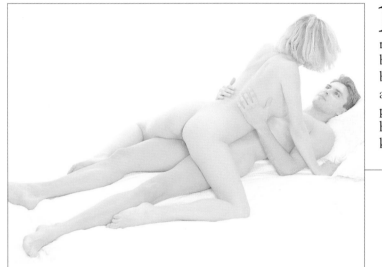

1 The woman starts from lying directly on top of her man. She then lifts herself up, brings her legs forward, and bends her knees. Initially, to avoid painful pressure on her partner, she will put most of her weight on her arms and knees.

2 By taking all her weight on her knees, she is free to use her hands on her partner — caressing him or holding him down to add an extra element of control, if she so wishes.

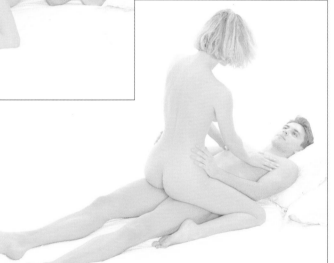

3 Or she can lean backward, pulling her legs behind and pressing them close to or pushing them away from her partner's body as she chooses. She even can bring her legs forward, stretching them toward her partner's shoulders. In this way, she is free to make swaying or rotating movements.

She can lean back onto his thighs to take some of her weight from his pelvis

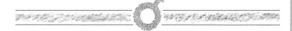

FOR THE MAN
These positions can be very exciting. The man has a full view of both his own and his partner's genitals, along with access to her breasts, and he is free to stimulate her and vice versa.

FOR THE WOMAN
In these positions a woman's breasts and genitals are free to be caressed, and she can most easily control the depth of penetration of her partner's penis.

He uses his hands to caress her bottom and to control the tempo and force of her movements

With all her weight on her knees, she can move freely and control the depth and position of her partner's penis

WOMAN-ON-TOP POSITIONS 3

Being on top puts the woman in control when making love, and if she adopts positions in which she faces away from her partner, she can more easily achieve the amount and type of stimulation she needs. For example, she can fantasize more freely if her partner is not in view, and she can reach down and stimulate herself without him seeing so there is no need for her to feel shy. Such positions, too, provide novel sensations for the woman that cannot be achieved any other way. For the man, such positions show that his partner is inventive at lovemaking. And if he is, as many men are, bottom-centered, when she kneels over him, displaying her thighs and buttocks in an enticing way, he will find such positions highly pleasurable.

Woman sitting forward
Here, the woman can use her hands to push off so she can raise or lower herself at will, gauging from her man's responses what he likes best. The position is very restful and stress-free for the man. He can, if he likes, bend his legs to offer support to his partner.

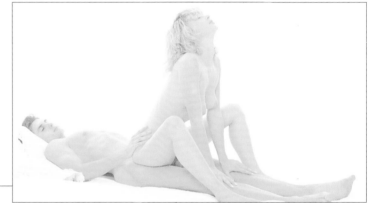

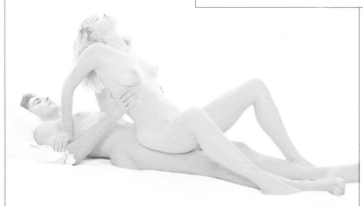

Woman stretched backward
In leaning back, the woman alters the depth of penetration and the sensations experienced. Now, most of her weight is directed at her feet, and her partner will find it uncomfortable if she presses too hard on his arms. This position gives him back some control over her movements. Care must be taken that the penis is not bent back at a painful angle.

FOR THE MAN
These positions give rein to a man's fantasies of having his penis used by his partner in the ways she wants. The loss of face-to-face contact can heighten his excitement if he lets his imagination conjure up for him those sexual situations that bring about the greatest arousal.

Woman with legs bent behind

Here, the woman sits forward again, giving her partner a good view of her buttocks. With her legs bent against him, he is in more control of her movements as she moves up and down on him. He can grasp her buttocks and encourage more vigorous movements or hold them back.

In this position she can move freely up and down on him

If she likes, she can turn to establish eye contact

She can move her hands forward to grasp his thighs and take some of her weight from her pelvis

He uses his hands to caress her bottom and to control the tempo and force of her movements

FOR THE WOMAN

Taking the active role enables a woman to give free rein to her fantasies and to achieve the type of stimulation she needs. In taking control of intercourse she becomes the active partner, and is free to make the movements that excite her most.

SITTING POSITIONS 1

Many couples find sitting positions extremely erotic — partly because of their novelty and partly because they are very intimate and allow close embraces. Sitting positions don't permit much movement or genital stimulation but they are restful and can be used when couples want to dampen their sexual ardor slightly before attempting further active love play.

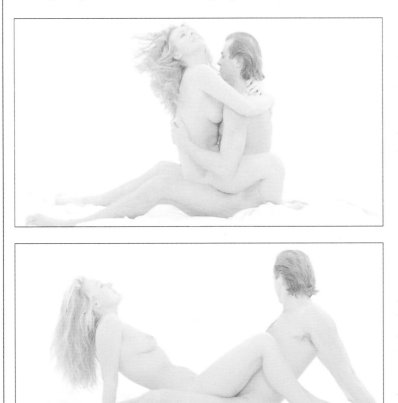

1 Couples can assume this position directly or convert from a woman-on-top position while the penis remains inside. This is achieved by the woman drawing her knees up under her so that she crouches over her partner. He should then straighten himself and support his body against his partner's while she slips her legs behind his back.

2 Finally, both partners can lean back, open their thighs, and enjoy the vision of their genital organs in union, which contributes significantly to sexual excitement. If the man initially inserts his penis in this position, his partner's hips should overlie his.

FOR THE MAN
These positions are not very tiring but they also don't allow much intense stimulation. Intimacy must bring its own excitement.

FOR THE WOMAN
These positions provide a great deal of intimacy and eye contact. Contracting her pelvic muscles increases the sensations for both.

3 In this position, the couple can indulge in close embraces, but genital stimulation is practically impossible unless the man stretches his arms behind him and thrusts himself forward.

The couple can kiss and embrace each other passionately, enjoying extreme intimacy

She can sit in his lap, his penis inside her, both enjoying tenderness but little physiological stimulation

He can raise and lower his knee to alter sensations

SITTING POSITIONS 2

Making love sitting down in a chair is a technique used by many couples, especially when they are having a "quickie," as only a minimal amount of undressing and preparation is required. They are also good where the man has some limitation of movement, due to illness, for example. Choose a sturdy, comfortable chair. If it has rungs, the woman can use them to support her feet and give her leverage to push against if she wants to move.

Woman sitting facing forward
If the woman sits facing her partner intense stimulation becomes possible. Here the woman can close her legs so that her vagina produces great pressure on the penis, and consequently greater sensation for both partners. If the man opens his thighs, the woman can push her body closer and his penis will extend further into her.

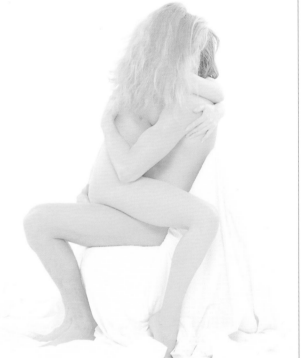

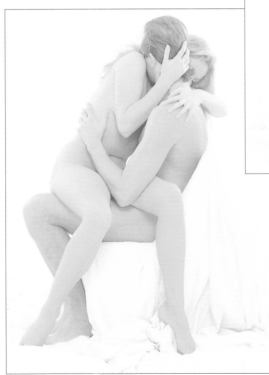

Woman sitting to the side
By turning to the side, the woman's genital area becomes available for manual stimulation by herself or her partner. She can still maintain her internal hold on the penis, and control its depth of penetration, but her sensations are likely to change.

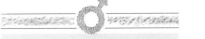

FOR THE MAN

Basically low energy, these positions allow the man to achieve great intimacy with his partner with little effort being expended. At the same time, they also are useful when time is short.

FOR THE WOMAN

These positions allow for a good deal of body and genital stimulation, and they also enable her to set the pace. Sitting positions are good variations when in a hurry or desirous of a change.

He can freely caress his partner's breasts and body, increasing her sensation and his own

She can use her hands to push off from her partner's knees

Woman sitting forward
Here the woman sits facing away from her partner with her feet supported on the floor so she bears some of her weight. Her partner is prevented from moving too much, so it is up to her to set the sexual tempo.

She can set the sexual pace, raising and lowering her hips off and on his penis

Having her feet on the floor can help balance when moving around in his lap

KNEELING POSITIONS 1

Throughout a lovemaking session, various postures should be adopted, both to vary the pace and sensation and, since intercourse can be strenuous, to rest or rejuvenate various bodily parts. Kneeling positions arise naturally out of man-on-top, woman-on-top, and standing positions, and can be usefully alternated with them or directly initiated. Kneeling positions are extremely arousing to the man as he gets a strong stimulus seeing his partner's body arched and open. For the woman, these positions can produce intense orgasms because they cause her to flex her internal muscles, which greatly increases sexual excitement for both partners.

He supports her weight on his bent legs and by grabbing her under the buttocks can pull her onto his erect penis

2 It is possible also for a supple woman to initate the position by arching her body, opening her legs, and offering her upraised vagina for the man to enter. The man must keep his hands under her hips to support her.

Both can maintain good eye contact and have the excitement of watching each other's bodies making love

She arches her back so that her pelvis is raised and open for him

1 The easiest position to assume is for the man to enter his partner from a man-on-top position. He should sit up, bringing his legs forward, and then place his partner's legs over his hips to raise her up slightly. Or, if the woman is sufficiently athletic, both partners can start in a kneeling position, and she can let herself slip backward.

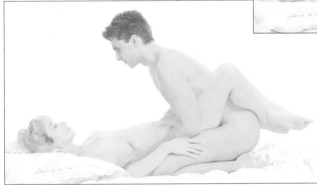

3 Finally, the man can kneel down, pulling his partner onto his thighs. She can twine her legs around him to add to his excitement. This maintains a good angle for penetration and gives him full view of their engaged genital organs, which is highly exciting and, at the same time, takes the strain off his back.

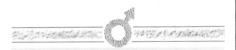

FOR THE MAN
As long as there are no back problems, these are useful positions that allow a good deal of movement and penetration. They offer much visual stimulation.

She uses her bent legs to raise herself toward her partner

FOR THE WOMAN
In most of these positions, the woman is manipulated by her partner; this can be appealing if she doesn't want to take too active a part. There is also plenty of opportunity for face-to-face contact.

KNEELING POSITIONS 2

Kneeling positions are more athletic than some, as they often involve lifting, but they are very versatile. Well-known variations include using chairs and sofas for support, as well as beds. The ones shown here are all frontal, or face-to-face, positions, but several of the rear-entry positions can also be carried out kneeling (see pages 138 to 141). Women, of course, can also play the dominant role and, in addition to the position shown below, several other kneeling ones are included in woman-on-top positions illustrated on pages 112 to 117.

Woman on top
A more athletic position, with plenty of body contact but giving the woman control over penetration, necessitates both partners squatting. This can prove to be tiring if carried on too long, and shouldn't be attempted by anyone with back or knee problems.

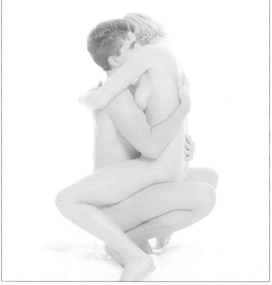

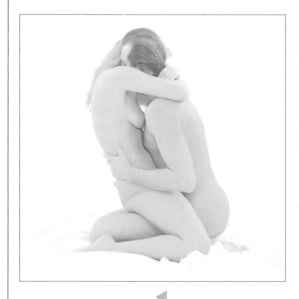

Upright variation
To assume this position both partners kneel on a soft surface. The woman spreads her thighs and either slides forward until her partner's knees are between her thighs, or she waits while her partner draws himself toward her.

FOR THE MAN
As long as he is as big or bigger than his partner, good stimulation of the woman's genitals is guaranteed, even when the penis is not fully erect.

FOR THE WOMAN
These positions can inject some variety into usual lovemaking practices. They are good because they enable the penis to directly stimulate the clitoris and vaginal lips.

Woman bent backward

Starting from a face-to-face position, with the woman bending slightly forward, the man inserts his penis into the vagina. Then he draws his partner up on him, so that her weight is supported by his arm under her buttocks, and leans over her. She can hold out her arm for support behind her.

She uses one arm to hold onto her partner so she can press against him

Using his arm to support her, he grasps her under the buttocks

He takes most of their combined weight on his knees

She transfers some of her weight to her hand so her partner can move her closer to him

KNEELING POSITIONS 3

With sufficient support, kneeling positions can be made more comfortable, and by raising or lowering the position of the woman's body, the man can adjust his approach to her vagina. This is a great advantage, and particularly useful in situations where a couple otherwise cannot achieve sufficient friction between the penis and vaginal walls. However, it is important in these variations to avoid very violent thrusts. If the man loses control he may propel his partner away from himself, or push her too hard against any support.

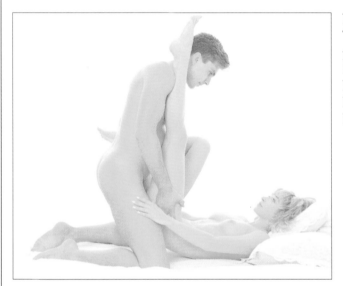

Legs held high
The man kneels by his recumbent partner, raising her legs above his hip level, and thrusts downward. From here, he also can manually stimulate her clitoris and reach forward to caress her breasts.

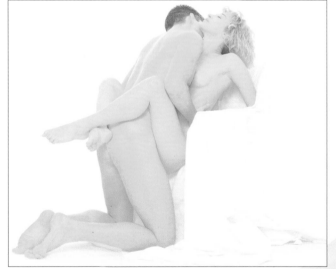

Woman raised high
Here the woman supports herself against a couch or chair while her partner kneels in front. Or, in a similar maneuver, she can lie on a table while her partner stands in front. She can recline and enjoy the sensations.

Genitals parallel
This comfortable position allows unhindered access to the penis, as well as permitting both partners to stimulate the clitoris and breasts. If the man gets tired of kneeling, they can alter the position by the woman pressing her thighs together while the man leans forward over her.

He can freely caress his partner's breasts and clitoris, and have the excitement of seeing her whole body while making love

He can control the depth of penetration by adjusting his partner's position to be closer or further away

She can recline comfortably on the bed, her hips just on the edge so that her vagina is easily accessible to her partner

FOR THE MAN
Much visual excitement is available from these postures and all allow for direct stimulation of the woman's genitals. They are good, too, for controlling ejaculation.

FOR THE WOMAN
These are more relaxing kneeling positions, during which the woman is free to stimulate herself if she so wishes. Or, she can be more active by leaning into her partner.

STANDING POSITIONS 1

Making love standing up is most achievable when both partners are about the same size. If the man is considerably larger than his partner, insertion and intercourse are only possible with a certain amount of difficulty. Sexual intercourse standing up can be tiring if kept up for any length of time, but because of the muscular exertion it necessitates, it can considerably increase sexual excitement.

   If the man picks up his partner, the greatest amount of exertion is the initial lift. Once he has achieved this, the position is not particularly tiring because the load is distributed between the two partners. From here, making love can continue while standing up, walking, or even dancing.

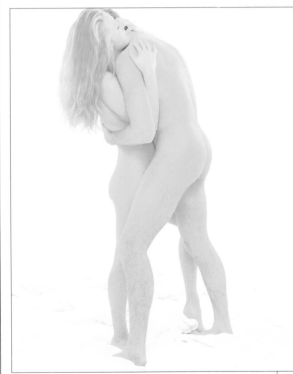

1 To facilitate insertion, the woman should lift one leg, turn it sideways so that her partner can introduce his penis, and then use both legs for support. The vagina clasps the penis firmly; she can use her pelvis to make strong sexual movements.

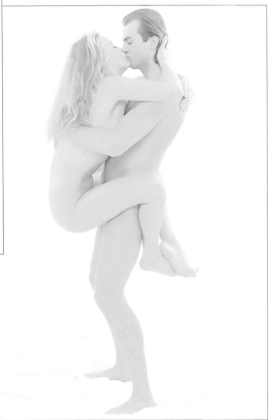

2 Once the man is inside, he can lift his partner by placing his hands under her thighs while she holds on to his neck. She should then cross her legs behind his back and press her thighs around his hips.

She can entwine herself around his body, gripping with her arms and thighs to distribute some of her weight. Her muscle tension can heighten sexual excitement for both of them

3 If both partners are agile, insertion can be achieved after the woman has been raised. Now the man can move his partner back and forth with his hands and alter tempo and motion.

FOR THE MAN
The main benefit of these positions is their novelty, since a good deal of agility and strength are required, but they are ideal when the man wants to dispense with preliminaries. More vigorous thrusts can be achieved if the woman is pressed against a wall or door for support.

FOR THE WOMAN
These positions are useful when the time and place for sex is limited, and when she wants to add some variety to her sex life. She can produce a very strong stimulation on her vaginal lips and clitoris by leaning forward a little and bending her knees while her feet are on the floor.

Grasping her under the buttocks, he can support her but also control the tempo of their lovemaking

With his legs bent, he can freely thrust into his partner

STANDING POSITIONS 2

It is even more important for partners to be of the same size when they attempt standing intercourse with the man inserting his penis from the back. While such positions are good for the man, in terms of freedom of movement and thrust, the woman's movements are fairly restricted and intimacy is, too. However, the act of being taken from behind is very exciting to the majority of women, and the back wall of the vagina can receive welcome stimulation.

1 If the man is taller than his partner, she can help him by bending forward a little and lifting her leg sideways. He can also bend slightly. Once he is inside, she can extend her leg again and straighten up.

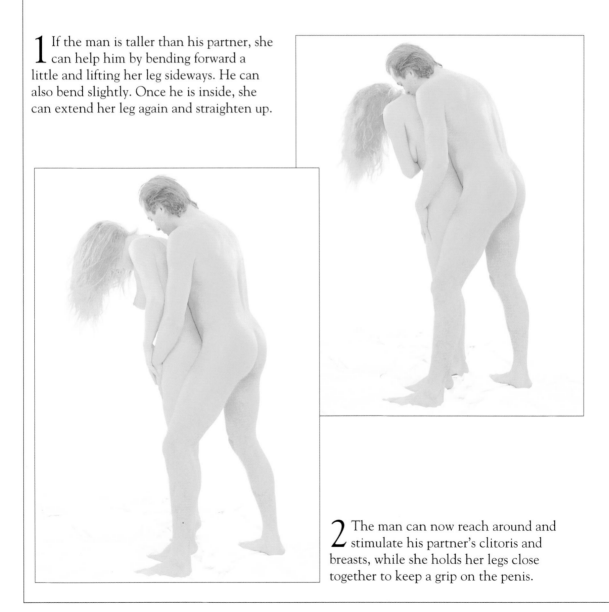

2 The man can now reach around and stimulate his partner's clitoris and breasts, while she holds her legs close together to keep a grip on the penis.

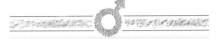

FOR THE MAN

These allow full stroke movement, deep penetration, and
access to his partner's clitoris.

FOR THE WOMAN

These are good for stimulating
the back of the vaginal walls,
which can lead to orgasms in
some inexperienced women.

Grasping her pelvis in his
hands, he can thrust
strongly into her, stimulating the rear vaginal wall and
thus increasing her chances
of orgasm

3 If the woman bends over,
holding on to her partner
for support, this greatly
facilitates the entry of the
penis into the vagina. The
man can grasp his partner's
buttocks with both hands as
he makes strong thrusting
movements with his hips. In
this way he can achieve
maximum penetration.

Her bending straight over
can facilitate maximum
penetration and full stroke
movement, producing deep
stimulation for them both

A solid footing is best,
but either partner can
stand on something
additional to increase
height, or crouch
slightly

SIDE-BY-SIDE POSITIONS 1

For relaxed, unhurried lovemaking, few positions beat side-by-side ones; it is not at all unusual for couples to fall asleep locked together after making love this way. When both people are on their sides, rear entry is easy, and intercourse can be prolonged easily, too, without being tiring. Such positions also provide maximum body contact and plenty of scope for caresses.

During pregnancy, and where a man is particularly large, side-by-side positions with the woman facing away are ideal. This way he can't put pressure on her. They also make a change from more athletic sexual postures.

1 The "spoons" position, with the man cuddling up to the woman's back, is one of the most comfortable and affectionate of all sexual positions. If the woman draws her knees upward, when her partner tucks up against her he can penetrate very easily.

Surrounding her body with his own, he can lovingly kiss and caress her back and neck, and reach around to stimulate her breasts and clitoris

Through the touch of his skin surrounding her, she can feel total intimacy in this gentle, relaxed lovemaking position

2 By moving onto her back a little more and raising her bottom slightly, her partner can thrust into her without restriction while having access to her breasts and vagina. There is a lot of skin contact, and the couple can kiss easily and passionately.

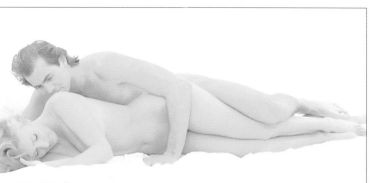

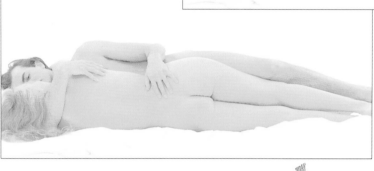

Facing variation
This can be achieved from a man-on-top position without disturbing intercourse, if both partners slide onto their sides. Or it can be initiated this way if the woman lifts or bends her leg to allow the man to insert his penis.

Raising her knee slightly allows him to penetrate her easily. Both partners are comfortable and can prolong their lovemaking for some time

FOR THE MAN

In these positions it is possible to achieve both maximum body contact and deep penetration. The man can reach around and touch his partner's breasts, vulva, clitoris, stomach, back, and neck.

FOR THE WOMAN

These positions are ideal for intimacy because they provide a lot of skin-to-skin contact. The opportunity for intimate conversation, caresses, and kisses make them sensual and romantic.

SIDE-BY-SIDE POSITIONS 2

By slight alterations in movement, side-by-side positions can produce a wide variety of new sensations. By rolling backward a woman opens up her vulva considerably and leaves her clitoris free for herself or her partner to caress. Drawing her legs upward increases penetration. By changing the position of his legs and thighs, the man can achieve different movements and control the pressure that the root of the penis directs against his partner's vulva.

Drawing her legs up along her partner's back and sides can increase penetration, particularly if she presses with her legs and feet, coaxing him to thrust further into her

1 The woman places her bent leg on top of her partner's hip as he pushes his thigh between hers. Then she should lie back and her partner can lean into her, keeping his legs stretched out straight. One of his arms is free to caress her, while she has both free to attend to him. He has more freedom to attempt active movements while bestowing some caresses.

FOR THE MAN

These positions give him good body contact with his partner and sufficient freedom to experiment with various movements to produce new sensations. While movement is somewhat limited, he is free to grasp his partner's buttocks and pull her onto his penis.

FOR THE WOMAN

These positions can supply plenty of pressure to the vulva for increased stimulation. They also are good during pregnancy as they allow a woman plenty of space from her partner, and his penetrating and thrusting movements can be restricted.

2 By bringing his leg back up, the man can now make strong pushing movements. He can increase the pressure by using his hands to press his partner's buttocks closer to his hips.

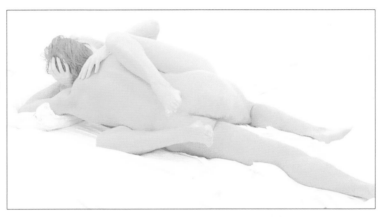

Changing the position of his legs and thighs can enable him to achieve different thrusting movements and new sensations for them both

SIDE-BY-SIDE POSITIONS 3

Side-by-side positions, because they are so comfortable, encourage experimentation even in couples who are unsure of each other or themselves: for example, a couple just beginning a sexual relationship. Variations on side-by-side positions offer full penetration with slight movement (which is good for the man who wants to control his orgasm), plus plenty of opportunity for passionate kissing and caressing. Women find them pleasurable, not least because they provide stimulation of the G spot, and some who have trouble experiencing orgasms find that these positions may help them to achieve them.

Both partners can maintain full eye contact and are free to engage in psssionate kissing

1 The man starts out lying curled up close to his partner with her knees over his thighs. From here he can reach down and insert his penis into her vagina in a gentle way. She should keep her legs closed tightly to hold his penis inside.

He uses his partner's body to push against for greater thrust

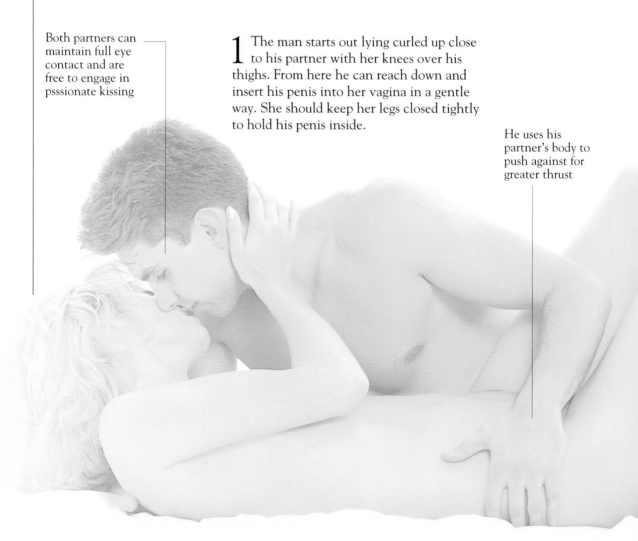

2 If the woman allows one leg to fall back, and the man brings his thigh over hers, this opens her vulva to more stimulation, and the pressure of the man's thigh on hers creates a warm, intimate sensation.

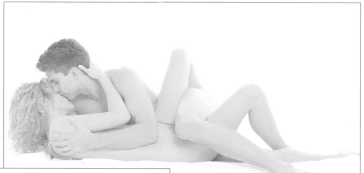

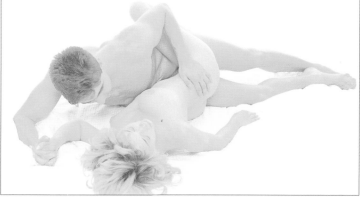

3 If both partners are a little athletic and want some variation, the woman should angle away from her partner, raising one knee. He can use it to push against and adjust his position so they achieve maximum genital contact.

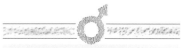

She can move her legs to alter the angle between vagina and penis

FOR THE MAN

Ideal when having sex with a new partner, they allow a wide range of passionate caresses and intimate conversation that can be carried out before, during, and after the penis is inserted.

FOR THE WOMAN

These comfortable and intimate postions can lead to a variety of sexual advances that are tender and non-threatening. Very often, too, they are blissfully sleep-inducing.

REAR-ENTRY POSITIONS

Although not as popular or as romantic as face-to-face positions, couples who have frequent intercourse enjoy the variety that a change to a rear-entry position can bring. Rear-entry positions provide the man with considerable freedom to thrust, and with them he can easily alter the angle and amount of penile movements. For women who have sensitive G spots, these positions result in the greatest stimulation; for those who don't, the different sensations produced still can be extremely exciting.

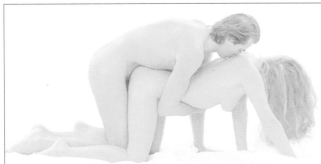

1 Probably the best-known and most widely used rear-entry position is known colloquially as the "doggie." To assume it, the woman kneels on her hands and knees on the bed or floor, and her partner kneels behind.

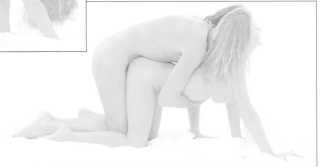

2 In this position, the vagina is turned straight back to the man pressed against her, and she can angle her pelvis in several different ways to give different sensations to both. Moreover, she can sway back and forth on her hands and knees.

3 The woman will find it more restful to slide down gently onto her stomach and chest while the man takes most of his weight on his hands. (The position can also be initiated in this way.) Deeper penetration will be achieved if she raises her bottom off the bed.

This position can be very exciting for a woman, if she is lithe enough, as excitement mounts from her partner's penis rubbing against new areas of her vagina that are not normally stimulated

4 By lying flat and pressing her legs together, the woman's clitoris and inner lips will be stimulated indirectly, maintaining her pleasure, and her partner can remain inside, moving as he pleases to rekindle desire.

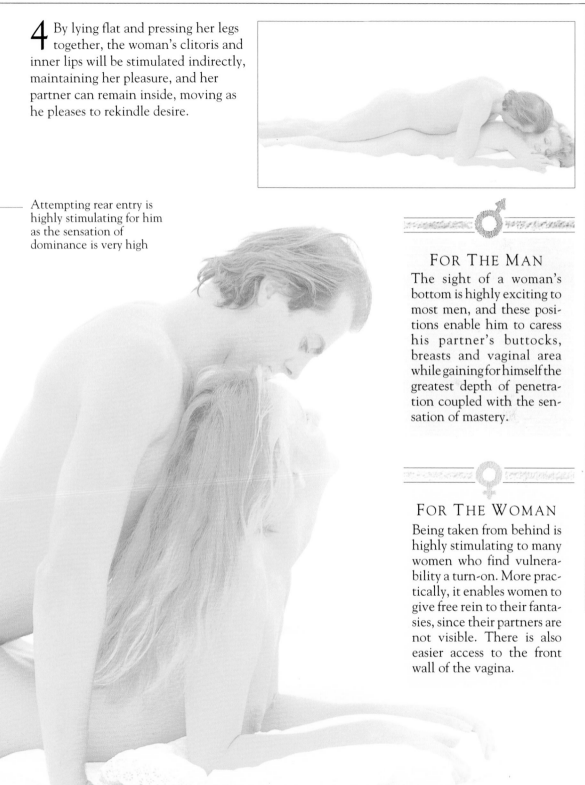

Attempting rear entry is highly stimulating for him as the sensation of dominance is very high

FOR THE MAN

The sight of a woman's bottom is highly exciting to most men, and these positions enable him to caress his partner's buttocks, breasts and vaginal area while gaining for himself the greatest depth of penetration coupled with the sensation of mastery.

FOR THE WOMAN

Being taken from behind is highly stimulating to many women who find vulnerability a turn-on. More practically, it enables women to give free rein to their fantasies, since their partners are not visible. There is also easier access to the front wall of the vagina.

REAR-ENTRY POSITIONS

Rear-entry positions can be somewhat athletic and are most preferred by adventurous lovers. Because of this, it is important that both partners feel comfortable; otherwise, if either finds a chosen position awkward, painful, or tiring, his or her lovemaking will naturally not be completely enjoyable, and the particular partner involved may feel coerced — a situation to be avoided.

In these positions women feel particularly vulnerable; for some this is exciting, for others it is not. Therefore, it is important that a man be sensitive to his partner's feelings and approach her with as much tenderness as the positions allow.

Upright "doggie" variation
A less submissive posture is when the woman kneels by the side of the bed, and her partner kneels behind her. As she leans over the bed and opens her legs, her partner enters her from behind. Now he can reach over and touch her breasts, and easily communicate his excitement and delight.

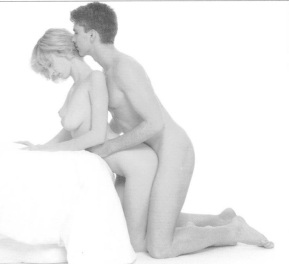

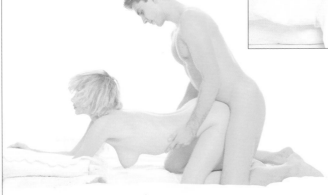

Woman inclining
This can be attempted with both the woman and man kneeling, or with the woman kneeling on a raised bed, her partner standing behind with his legs slightly bent. The woman should open her legs wide, to expose her upturned vagina. In this position, there is strong friction for the penis.

FOR THE MAN

Among the most exciting positions, they offer great depth of penetration. This makes them particularly good for men who have difficulty in inserting the penis into a partner's vagina.

FOR THE WOMAN

A great many unusual and exciting sensations can be experienced in these positions, but to avoid any discomfort or fear, she should communicate her feelings to her partner.

Woman on top
The man sits up and the woman crouches over him, her back to his face. Then he lowers his partner onto his penis; this gives him exceptional penetration. The woman, however, must push herself up and down to create thrusting, or she can contract her pelvic muscles for stimulation.

She can take her weight on her hands and feet and use them to raise and lower herself at will

He uses his hands to guide and control his partner's movements

MORE ADVANCED POSITIONS

While a couple often has reservations about changing established patterns of love-making to incorporate more unusual positions, a little experimentation can do much to enliven one's sex life and bring new and exciting sensations.

Sexual athletics for their own sake have little to recommend them, but making love in the same positions year after year can prove equally unsatisfactory. A couple needs to experiment to find out which positions give them the best sensations, and some of the more exotic positions are exactly those that meet a couple's specific needs. It isn't necessary for couples to indulge in these more fanciful positions on a regular basis, unless they find them particularly rewarding, but for special occasions they are worth a try.

One thing to bear in mind, however, is that these positions by and large demand that partners be supple and athletic, and that they don't differ too much in size.

FOR THE MAN
Variety is the spice of life and a jaded appetite or flagging sexual drive can be improved by trying something new.

FOR THE WOMAN
Some highly unusual positions provide stimulation in parts of the vagina no others can, and for this sake should be tried.

Man facing away
The woman lies down with her legs up, open, and wide apart. The man lowers himself onto her from an outward-facing position. He penetrates her in reverse, and from here can make thrusting movements. She can reach down and feel his testicles, buttocks, and anus.

She can caress her partner's buttocks and testicles

Pillows or heaped bedding will make her position more comfortable

Backward woman-on-top

With the man lying on his back, the woman kneels down with her back to his face and lowers herself on his erect penis. Then she leans back as far as she can. Here she receives stimulation on the front wall of her vagina, and her breasts and clitoris can be manually stimulated.

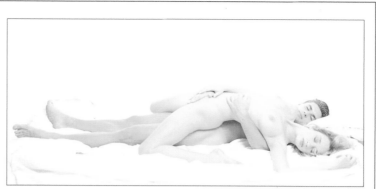

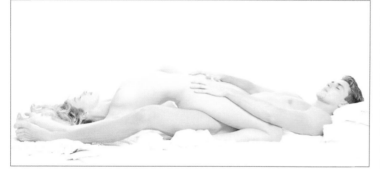

Lean-back variation

The woman starts from an on-top position facing her partner, then gradually, very gently, leans backward until her head is flat down. Now she receives pleasant and unusual sensations on the vagina's front wall. She can also stretch her legs out in front to vary her sensations.

He assumes an essentially restful pose but novel sensations are achieved by thrusting backward

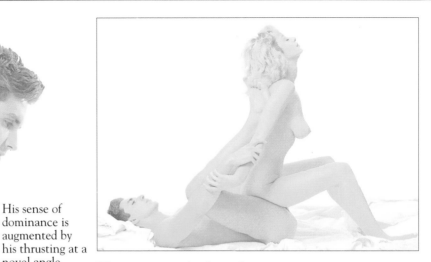

His sense of dominance is augmented by his thrusting at a novel angle producing new sensations

Woman sitting backward
The man lies on his back and pulls his knees to his chest. The woman then lowers herself onto his penis, easing him inside her. She can lean back against his legs for support, while he steadies her using his hands.

She should support herself on the bedding. A woman should never attempt this if she is pregnant or has a weak back

She finds this position very exciting, if she is lithe enough, since his penis rubbing against areas of her vagina not normally stimulated results in new sensations

Woman bent over
The woman can either assume this head-down position before the man penetrates her, or bend down once he has entered her from a standing position.

ANAL PENETRATION

Anal intercourse — penis in rectum — is often a homosexual activity, although heterosexual couples occasionally practice it since it can evoke highly erotic responses. Men, when they will admit it, also like to be penetrated and, particularly when the woman has had several children, the anus offers a pleasant tightness. Moreover, if the woman has her partner at her rear, he can stimulate her breasts, clitoris and vagina more easily.

Men are nearly always the initiators, as the vast majority of women rate it as their least favorite sexual activity. Some men introduce the activity as a way of expanding a couple's sexual repertoire, and some women respond enthusiastically. Unfortunately, however, other men use demands for anal sex as a way of testing a relationship, and this is never a good reason for having it.

THE AIDS CONNECTION

Anal sex has been implicated in the spread of the HIV virus, the causative factor in AIDS; it is far riskier for unprotected couples than vaginal sex, and should never be undertaken with casual, occasional partners. Only if you have anal sex with one regular partner *and* you are both faithful to each other *and* neither of you are HIV-positive, can you be certain of not contracting AIDS. Of course, a condom should be used, but this does not guarantee safety.

Other germs also can be transferred from the anus to the vagina, which can cause infections. If the penis has been inserted in the anus it must be thoroughly washed immediately afterward.

If anal sex is to be undertaken, it is important to recognize that the anus was not anatomically designed for intercourse, and infections and injuries can result even with the gentlest lover. Practiced regularly for a long time, control of the anal sphincter may be lost and incontinence can result.

When planning to indulge in this type of penetration, it is a good idea to build up to it gradually. Over a period of time, partners should try some of the techniques of anal stimulation (see page 90) before attempting full penetration.

Once both partners are ready, the man always must be well lubricated and should insert himself slowly and gently. The man should stop penetration immediately if he is asked, since anal intercourse can be very painful for his partner. The woman can help by adopting an on-top rear-entry position, and relaxing her anal sphincter as much as she can by bearing down slightly. Penetration is not normally very deep, about an inch on the first few attempts.

AFTERPLAY

On all levels — physical, emotional, and mental — men and women experience the period of resolution in different ways. While both feel relaxed, calm, and satisfied, they have experienced a type of communion which is ecstatic and timeless. Then they return to the normal world and become aware of their surroundings. A man does this much more quickly than a woman. Detumescence is very fast; the penis becomes flaccid within a minute. A woman takes much longer to surface from the depths of her orgasm, especially if her experience was intense. The engorgement of her genital organs resolves much more slowly, and so do her emotions.

Most women wish to stay in an embrace while their partners want to get up, have a cigarette, or simply go to sleep. This is a classic instance of why it is important for partners to talk about their desires and to reach a happy solution. If they don't, the situation can lead to unhappiness, frustration, and resentment.

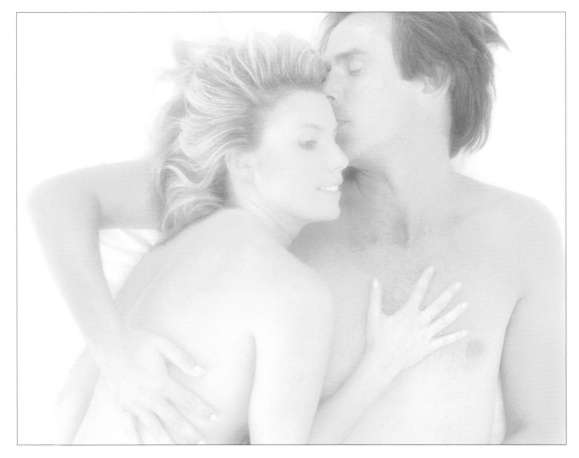

THE MAN'S EXPERIENCE

Once a man has ejaculated, his interest in sex, and possibly his partner, declines rapidly. His penis will shrink and his sex drive departs. For a period of time, mainly depending upon his age and health, he won't be able to achieve another erection, and therefore, his interest in sex is lessened.

For many men, the penis becomes extremely sensitive immediately after orgasm, necessitating instant withdrawal from the vagina. Such men will withdraw physically from their partners, moving and turning away from them.

In addition, many men may be overcome by postcoital somnolence. During the arousal period, a large amount of blood flows into the man's pelvic area, and his muscles contract and tighten. This blood is rapidly diverted away from the area after sex, and his muscles relax so that excitement is replaced by drowsiness and a general feeling of lethargy — something not experienced by the majority of women. Often a man will roll over to his side of the bed and go to sleep, leaving his partner in the "wet spot."

— ACCOMMODATING A PARTNER —

The majority of men are completely unaware of how a woman interprets these movements. After orgasm, women experience no such feelings of hypersensitivity. During the slow phase of female detumescence, and still savoring the effects of an orgasm, most women feel the strong desire to remain entwined in a partner's arms and to lie quietly close to him, enjoying nonpassionate embraces and caresses.

Even if a man cannot combat his physiological reactions to orgasm, he can and should be sensitive to his partner's emotional needs. A last cuddle and good-night kiss can be bestowed before he drifts off without too much effort. A shift to lovemaking during the morning, when both partners are fresher, or during the day, may help to stave off sleep.

THE WOMAN'S EXPERIENCE

During the slow phase of female detumescence, while still savoring the effects of an orgasm, most women feel the strong desire to remain entwined in their partners' arms, and to lie quietly close to them enjoying nonpassionate embraces and caresses. Some will even wish to lie with their partner's penis still inside them, flaccid though they may be.

Usually women wish to maintain a close embrace; they are quite prepared to lie for a long time, totally relaxed but in full embrace with their partners on top or between their legs. There is a theory that a woman's instinct for sexual pleasure is so deeply ingrained in her nature that she has an overwhelming need to maintain body contact with her partner after orgasm, and thereby extend the period of enchantment for as long as possible.

But if her partner gets up or simply rolls over and goes to sleep, a women feels neglected and bereft, and this kind of turning off without explanation after sexual union usually leaves her feeling lonely. A sudden withdrawal of this kind seems uncaring, if not brutal, to her.

— PROLONGING A MAN'S INTEREST —

A man's normal physiological response to orgasm is one of drowsiness and lethargy, and this is enhanced if lovemaking is done at times when he is already feeling tired and ready for sleep. Therefore, a change to morning lovemaking may bring about more affectionate afterplay.

To encourage your partner to stay awake, keep conversation light and romantic; tell him how much you love him and how wonderful he is. It is a good idea to avoid talking about household problems, as this is certain to send him to sleep. Make sure, too, that after having sex it is not you who rushes off immediately to the bathroom to wash. If you must wash yourself, suggest taking a bath together.

THE FIRST SEXUAL EXPERIENCE

The driving force behind your first sexual experience may be love, but it could also be lust, or even curiosity. It is quite usual for most people to be a little apprehensive and tense, and also to feel a little disappointed with the outcome — first-time sex might not prove to be the ecstatic experience they had imagined. Like most things, sex invariably improves with practice and familiarity with your partner. While for most men, orgasm is fairly automatic even on the first occasion, women rarely achieve orgasm with early intercourse; this is something that has to be learned.

MAKING IT BETTER

It will certainly help, however, if you choose the right setting and make sure you have complete privacy with no fear of interruptions. You should decide beforehand whether you will be spending the night together or leaving before morning. If the former, you not only need to think about bringing a change of clothes, but how you will feel about waking up with someone you might not know very well.

Allow yourselves plenty of time so that your lovemaking can proceed unhurried. With the first time this is especially important, since any nervousness that one or both partners feel must be completely dispelled if arousal is to take place. The man particularly should not be in too much of a hurry.

Make sure a reliable form of contraception is used. Lovers should bear in mind, too, that as AIDS and other sexually transmitted diseases can be caught or spread the first time sexual intercourse takes place, the man should also wear a condom (see Safe Sex, page 244).

Virgins should declare themselves; this is particularly important for the woman, because she needs to inform her partner to be gentle and not to thrust too deeply at first. The man should make certain the woman is aroused by caressing and stimulating her for at least ten minutes before penetration. This way she will have enough natural lubrication to make things easier. In addition, saliva or artificial lubricants can be used to make things more comfortable.

Choose a man-on-top position; putting a pillow beneath the woman's hips may make it more comfortable for her. Penetration should be gentle but firm, and thrusts should be light. A woman can help her man by guiding his penis into her vagina, and bearing down slightly as he enters to relax the pelvic muscles.

Loving
Sex
Throughout
Life

ADAPTING SEX

In my opinion, sex is necessary for a contented life. It appeals to the intellect and the emotions like little else can. It makes us feel needed, wanted, secure, and desirable. Because good sex is so important to a healthy self-image, the brain would make us seek sex even if the physical needs of the body did not.

However, during a couple's lifetime, there are occasions when normal sexual practices may be interrupted. Nonetheless, there would appear to be no instance, as long as partners desire each other, in which all sexual intimacy would be prohibited.

WHEN ACTIVITIES MAY NEED ADJUSTING

During pregnancy, the frequency of intercourse may decline gradually, but a fair number of couples have intercourse more often and enjoy sex more than ever before, possibly because they are no longer worrying whether conception will occur. During pregnancy, a woman's body can respond more floridly to sexual arousal; all impulses and sensations become heightened due to the high levels of circulating sex hormones.

After the birth of a baby, there are no particular physical difficulties that preclude sexual intercourse, though it is normal for mothers, and even a number of fathers, not to feel like sex for several weeks, no matter how close and loving the couple had been before.

It is hard to imagine the disease that sexual intercourse is bad for. Research data indicates that the maximum heart rate during a typical workday is much higher than that achieved during orgasm, and blood pressure changes with sexual activity are not at the risk level. Your rule should be that unless your doctor says you should not have sex, you will probably benefit from sex, and not simply survive it.

Our feelings about love and sex do not change very much as we get older; they develop and, if anything, become stronger and more passionate, even more tender.

As a couple gets older, they come to see sexual contact and its frequency differently from their youth. To a loving couple, sexual union is an affirmation of something that goes beyond a moment's pleasure. Years of giving and receiving love strengthens their union. One contact a month may be fulfilling enough for many couples, reflecting as it does three, four, or five decades of intimacy.

There are many reasons why sex should remain good as we get older. There is more privacy and fewer interruptions, and many couples feel that they have reached a time in their lives where they can proceed more slowly and savor the best moments in sex.

SEX IN PREGNANCY

If a woman's pregnancy is proceeding normally, there is absolutely no reason why she and her partner should not enjoy full sexual relations right up until the time of labor. A woman's sex drive can vary in pregnancy, fluctuating up and down, but the majority of women state that sex during pregnancy is better than ever before. This is due to the high level of circulating sex hormones that in many women increase sex drive, making them more responsive to sex and their arousal rapid and full.

Some women experience a loss of libido during the first or third trimesters, often as the result of morning sickness at the beginning of pregnancy, and tiredness toward the end. In addition, no woman is particularly fond of her large shape, and this may make her feel embarrassed to undress and make love.

The breasts can be particularly sensitive and tender, and a partner should be gentle. As the fetus enlarges and occupies more of the abdominal and pelvic cavities, couples may find themselves spontaneously changing their techniques and their positions (see page 152). Old wives' tales say that sexual intercourse may cause an infection prior to labor that may affect the baby, but the uterus is completely sealed off by a mucus plug, so intercourse should not lead to an ascending infection as long as good sexual hygiene is practiced by both partners. However, a great deal of vigorous sexual activity might lead to abrasions and soreness and, where there is poor hygiene, it is conceivable that an infection could ensue. So, with the understanding that you have sex only with your partner, and only when you feel like it, and as long as it is not too athletic, sex is recommended throughout pregnancy unless your doctor advises otherwise.

Some women are scared that sex will crush the baby. This is not possible because the baby is suspended in the amniotic sac and surrounded by amniotic fluid, which cushions it from any kind of bumping and bruising.

WHEN NOT TO HAVE SEX

• If bleeding occurs, consult your doctor immediately. It may not be serious, but your doctor has to rule out possible placenta previa or a miscarriage.

• If you have a show (the appearance of blood-stained vaginal discharge which heralds the onset of labor) or your water breaks.

• If you have had a previous miscarriage, ask your doctor's advice; you may be advised to abstain during the early months while the pregnancy establishes itself.

• If your obstetrician advises you to abstain.

POSITIONS FOR PREGNANCY

Bodily changes caused by pregnancy may mean that intercourse will be more comfortable in certain positions. During the first few months, you probably won't have to alter your lovemaking at all, although if there has been a previous misarriage, you should avoid deep penetration. In the middle months, when a woman's abdomen has enlarged, rear-entry, side-by-side, and woman-on-top positions work well. In the latter months of pregnancy, with both her breasts and abdomen swollen, a woman will find that being approached from behind while on all fours, and some of the woman-on-top positions, are highly arousing and still comfortable.

The man uses his arm
to support his weight

Rear-entry positions
These can be used throughout pregnancy, although the woman may alter her position to accommodate the baby by changing from lying on her side to being on all fours.

She can take the weight off her abdomen
by rolling back on her hip

Side-by-side positions
A variation that is particularly suited to pregnancy, the woman can maneuver herself onto her partner's penis.

He can caress her freely, including
her genital area

She keeps her legs
close together in order
to grasp his penis

Sitting positions
These positions, with the woman sitting astride her partner, are most useful in the early and middle months. While they don't allow a lot of movement, they are comfortable for both partners and alleviate pressure on the abdomen so there is no fear of "crushing" the baby. Also, if deep penetration presents problems, here she can control the depth of penetration to a great extent.

She can adjust her position so she is comfortable and still able to caress him

Though his movements are limited, it is a very intimate position

She can rest some of her weight on her feet, taking the strain off her partner

SEX AFTER CHILDBIRTH

Sexual difficulties connected with childbirth are not uncommon. Many women suffer from anemia, extreme tiredness, or depression after pregnancy, and all of these lower sex drive. There may also be an injury from labor or hormonal disturbances. In the early weeks or months after childbirth, a woman may be completely involved with her new baby and her maternal energies, and she may be totally sapped by attending to the baby and going without sleep at night. This leaves very little energy for anything, including sex.

Men, too, are affected by childbirth. While some men enjoy being present at the birth of their child, others are so affected in the opposite way by the experience (especially if the birth has required medical intervention such as a Caesarean section or an episiotomy) that they avoid sex in an unconscious attempt to prevent their partner from having to go through such "horrors" again.

By far the greatest complaint is the aftereffects of an episiotomy — the cut made in the perineum to allow the baby's head to be born and to prevent tearing during delivery. An episiotomy scar is often painful and, particularly if it is large, can make sex so uncomfortable that women shrink even from an embrace that might lead to other sexual activities. Quite often women feel sexy, aroused, and ready for sexual union, but the scar hurts so much that penetration is impossible, often for up to six months after delivery.

WHEN TO RESUME RELATIONS

Even taking the above into account, it is a good idea for you to resume your sex life after only a brief interval. You should experiment, carefully and gently, to find out what kind of sexual enjoyment can be achieved together with your partner. You could practice sex that is nonpenetrative but nonetheless entirely fulfilling and satisfying within a few days of delivery, if you both feel like it.

Many women want to return to having orgasms a few days after birth, and having orgasms can be beneficial because it seems to help the uterus return to its normal state. There is no danger in attempting full sexual intercourse ten to 14 days after a vaginal delivery if the episiotomy is healed and discharge has stopped. (After a Caesarean section, wait four to six weeks to allow the uterus to heal.)

While it is quite normal for both partners not to feel like sex for some time after a birth, many couples do feel that it is a bad idea to put off sex indefinitely because abstinence becomes a habit. The first time may seem like an ordeal, but it is worth trying and speeds up the resumption of normal sexual relations.

SEX DURING ILLNESS

I don't believe that illness should preclude sex. Naturally, if either partner becomes seriously ill, then neither may even think about sex. But if the illness is long-term, it is unrealistic to expect both partners to forego the pleasure that sexual union brings. In the first place, you should take your doctor's advice, and if there is none against having sexual relations, then, by mutual consent, you can try exploring the possibilities. The type of illness and the seriousness of the sick person's condition must be borne in mind. Sex should not be too strenuous and positions not too demanding (see page 156). It is the responsibility of the partner who is well to make sure that the other is rested and relaxed and not only able to cope with sex, but desirous of it. It is also probably up to the healthy partner to initiate sex.

FACTORS THAT INHIBIT PERFORMANCE

Many drugs interfere with the sex drive and, in addition, can affect erections, ejaculation, and clitoral sensitivity. These medicines are many and varied, and are used for the treatment of anxiety, insomnia, obesity, asthma, tension, diabetes, and high blood pressure. They may, in certain people, adversely affect sexual performance.

This is also true of another drug: alcohol. Alcohol in the blood directly suppresses sexual reflexes and about half of all men suffering from alcoholism have problems with erection; a much higher proportion of women experience loss of sex drive.

After abdominal or pelvic surgery, it would be wise not to indulge in sexual intercourse for at least six to eight weeks, giving tissues time to heal and scars to become less sensitive. In the case of major surgery, recovery may take as long as three months before you feel you have enough energy and interest to cope with sex. But with any other type of surgery, it is largely up to you and your partner. If you are feeling well and relaxed, there is no reason why you and your partner should not enjoy gentle, exploratory sex whenever you feel like it, within a week of surgery if you are both feeling up to it. You must take things at your own pace, as dictated by your strength, mood, and inclination. Unless specifically advised by your doctor not to have sexual relations, however, follow your own instincts.

Some people, of course, will use surgery or an illness as an excuse and an explanation for not having sex, but you and your partner should be aware of the true motivation. Everyone can have a fulfilling sex life no matter what illness he or she may be suffering from. Remember that no disease or illness completely prevents us from making sexual contact with someone we love.

POSITIONS DURING ILLNESS

Depending upon your individual situation, positions need to be chosen carefully so that they produce pleasure without discomfort. To start with, the affected partner should do the least work, so if a man has been ill, choose a woman-on-top position, and if it is the woman who is affected, attempt a rear-entry position. Where both partners have limitations, side-by-side positions work well.

It is important, too, to choose positions where there is sufficient support for body parts, and very often a bed is not the best place for sex. Chairs, sofas, and tables may offer greater scope for successful sexual activity. Cushions and pillows can be employed strategically to raise or lower partners or cushion sensitive areas.

Man-on-top positions
This variation, with the woman lying fully supported, enables the man to have complete control over his thrusting, so that he penetrates her only to the depth and extent it is comfortable.

He can adjust the angle of his insertion so it is most comfortable

Her movement is extremely limited but there is no pressure on her body

Approaching on his knees means it is less tiring for him

Sitting positions

When the man is not able to take a more active part, these positions enable the woman to control the pace of lovemaking. With her back to her partner, he can reach around and caress her breasts while penetrating her in a gentle way.

While not able to make active thrusting movements, he can caress his partner's breasts and clitoris

She can bear some of her weight on her feet, and use them to move up and down

Rear-entry positions

This is a fairly comfortable position for the woman who can lean against the bed for support and cushion her knees with pillows. The man can concentrate his efforts on penetration, while being able to caress her breasts and clitoris.

She can rest her weight against the bed

HEART DISEASE AND SEX

Largely due to fear, fewer than one person in four returns to the sexuality he or she enjoyed before a heart attack. And yet all the news on heart disease is extremely good. Doctors now realize that a normal sex life can greatly benefit people who suffer heart attacks, and they encourage a return to normal sexual activity as soon as possible. It may be that the pattern of your sexual relationship has to change; most people with heart disease are very tired at the end of the day, but after a good night's sleep, when both partners are fresh, sex may seem more attractive. A change in position can also help (see page 156).

Avoid drinking alcohol and eating rich, heavy meals at night, since these both put a strain on the heart and any sexual activity would only add to the burden. If you do experience chest pains such as angina while you are having sex, ask your doctor about using one of the nitrate preparations which you can slip under the tongue whenever pain approaches, in exactly the same way as you would if you got pain when you were walking up a steep hill.

High blood pressure itself should not be a deterrent to sexual activity. Sex is not bad for high blood pressure; however, many of the drugs taken to treat high blood pressure may result in a loss of libido. Not all hypotensive agents have this side effect and, if you need treatment for high blood pressure, ask your doctor to prescribe a drug that does not affect sexual drive.

ARTHRITIS AND SEX

Arthritis can cause discomfort during sexual intercourse, and you may find that it affects your sex life. The ordinary face-to-face position can be made difficult by painful, stiff joints, but there is no reason why you should not try a new position — for example, with the woman on top if the man is arthritic. This is particularly useful in situations where the man experiences pain when he moves, or if it is difficult for him to bear weight on his arms, knees, or shoulders. Or you might try having the man sit in a chair or on the edge of the bed while the woman gently lowers herself onto him. The spoons position, with the man behind the woman, works for some.

You can ease the pain and stiffness in your joints by taking your painkilling drugs an hour or so before having sex. A warm bath is a pleasant prelude to making love, and helps to mobilize stiff joints. Even if the problems involved in making love are so restricting that you decide to forego full intercourse, there is no reason why you should abstain from other sexual activities if you and your partner would like them. Everyone gains comfort and reassurance from physical closeness through touching and caressing.

DIABETES AND SEX

Sexual disturbance is not necessarily a complication of diabetes mellitus, but it can interfere with long-term sexual contentment. If diabetes is not controlled it can cause impotence in men, creating difficulty in attaining both erections and ejaculations. Lower testosterone levels are probably the cause of male impotence, and may be caused by a malfunction of the nerves that supply the penis. Some men also complain of premature ejaculation. Even a temporary disturbance in sexual potency can cause men anxiety that may lead to further impotence.

Women diabetics are more prone to vaginal yeast infections, and this condition can cause local irritation and even pain during intercourse. They also may have difficulty with vaginal lubrication.

If you are suffering from these problems, you are not alone. Approximately half of all men who suffer from diabetes have problems with erection, although diabetes itself is not necessarily the cause; some of the drugs used for treatment can cause erection problems, so consult your doctor about possibly changing to another. Yeast infections are easily treated with modern fungicides.

Sexual problems and diabetes are not static and therefore the outlook is not a pessimistic one. Arousal, ejaculation, and orgasm vary from time to time and do improve, so don't give up sex altogether. Keep on trying it every now and then. Try to maintain a positive attitude so that you and your partner can experience a mutually pleasing sex life that may be different from the one you had before, but which is still fulfilling.

MULTIPLE SCLEROSIS AND SEX

Multiple sclerosis is an inflammation of the lining of the nerves due to an unknown cause. Inflammation is patchy and unpredictable, and it is impossible to know ahead of time which nerves will be affected. However, a quarter of all men with the disease might expect problems with erection due to inflammation of the nerves to the penis, and about the same number of women might suffer from the most common sexual complaint, a decrease of clitoral sensitivity.

Both sexes suffer a loss of libido, but the sex drive can vary greatly over time so it is important that partners of multiple sclerosis patients encourage intimacy. There is always the possibility that sex drive and other sex functions will return. Close physical contact will be maintained and a positive benefit achieved if the able partner helps the affected one into comfortable positions, which may be in places other than a bed.

SEX AFTER MASTECTOMY

Radical mastectomy, a brutal operation with a very disfiguring scar, is thankfully becoming a surgical technique of the past. Nonetheless, cancer of the breast may have to be treated by procedures that do leave disfigurement. Although reconstructive surgery is widely and successfully practiced, nearly all women who have any form of treatment for breast tumors confess to being more anxious about any scars that may result than about life expectancy. In our society, the sexuality of the breast has probably been overemphasized, leading women to feel denuded of their femininity if their breasts lose their shape and firmness. Many women suffer terrible insecurity, worrying that their partners will no longer find them sexually desirable. If only women would talk to their partners in these situations, they would be greatly reassured, because most partners of women who have had mastectomies state that their only concern is the well-being of their women. This overrides everything else, and most of them say that their sexual feelings for their partners are not impaired by the loss of one of their breasts.

Despite this, about one-third of women who have a mastectomy fail to resume sexual activity even six months after surgery. This must be due to a failure to communicate between couples, because over half the men and women in marriages where the wife has had a mastectomy feel an increased need for intimacy.

It helps a woman if she tries to see her body as a whole, rather than concentrating on the scar itself. When we look at another person's body we do not just look at one part, we take in the whole picture. Couples should attempt to do this as soon as possible after surgery. It helps if the normal breast is felt first when the man reaches for his partner, so, if necessary, partners should change the side of the bed they normally sleep on. You may have to change how you have sex, but this does not necessarily diminish it; indeed, it can be stimulating to concentrate on a new part of the body rather than the breasts.

DISABILITY AND SEX

The general attitude to people in wheelchairs and the physically handicapped or disabled is that all sexual possibilities are ruled out. Speak to such a person and you will find that this is entirely incorrect. For many couples, sex can be as good or better after a stroke or a disabling injury. People in this situation have no lack of sexual urge. What they lack is privacy; most people around them neglect to consider that they may feel like having sex in a perfectly normal way.

Because sex is never only genital, it can always be enjoyed by a disabled person. The inability to move, for instance, does not mean the inability to please. The absence of sensation does not mean the absence of feelings. A disabled person still feels desire; there is no loss of sexuality just because the genital organs do not function. The ability to enjoy persists even though the ability to perform does not. Loving, satisfying, and fulfilling sex is there for every couple to enjoy; they simply have to find it for themselves.

VARYING SEXUAL ACTIVITY TO ACHIEVE SATISFACTION

Some people who are handicapped can enjoy a nearly normal sex life with some variation of positioning for genital intercourse. For others, altered forms of sexual activity, or those of a noncoital nature such as touching, kissing, petting, or oral-genital stimulation, will be needed depending on the degree to which a partner or partners can move, how much pain there is, whether there are spasms, etc. Most importantly, communication must be open and plentiful so that partners can find out what needs to be done to achieve sexual satisfaction for both. The need to be more open and experimental can lead couples to discover a range of touching, positions, and pleasures that able-bodied couples may never discover.

Handicapped people should engage in any sexual activity that is physiologically possible, pleasurable, and acceptable to them. A priority is to find a comfortable position, and in this case using pillows and cushions may help to lend support to or take pressure off various areas. Problems with lubrication can be helped by using KY Jelly (not Vaseline, which can cause vaginal infections).

Even the possibility of urinary or bowel incontinence should not preclude sex. A catheter that can't be removed can be taped to the stomach or inner thigh to help keep it out of the way. An ileostomy bag, if it is firmly in place, can be left as is. It should be emptied before intercourse to avoid accidents, and then taped in place. Paraplegics, too, can be taught to stimulate their partners using hands, mouth, toes, a towel, etc., and to gain as much pleasure as possible from being touched themselves.

When there is no feeling in the sexual organs, often other parts of the body increase in sexual feeling and, in these circumstances, it is important for the person involved to understand his or her own body and communicate which areas are still sensitive to sexual arousal when stimulated. Orgasm can still be achieved even when a significant part of the body is without sensation or motion. Sexual satisfaction may even be completely nonphysical and may manifest itself as an emotional or spiritual release.

If you have a physical disability that is causing you serious personal problems, ask your doctor to refer you to a sex therapist.

SEX AND THE OLDER LOVER

I find it reassuring that the majority of older people still find sex thrilling and energy-giving; neither their desires or capabilities vanish. Sex may wane a little in frequency and vigor, but not in sweetness and satisfaction. Exactly as in relationships at a young age, attraction and love are followed by sexual desire and sexual fulfilment. The basic qualities in a relationship strengthen as we get older; they do not weaken.

There are many reasons why sex should remain good as we get older; we lose many of our inhibitions and we feel a need and a freedom to enjoy sexual pleasures that we would have kept hidden when we were younger. We may experience also a feeling that time is running out and we should do as we wish, as long as we do not hurt anyone. Incursions on our time and privacy, such as children and domestic chores, have been left behind, so there is more time and energy to be invested in sex. Most of us become somewhat more sophisticated in later life in controlling intimate situations, and therefore feel more at ease in them and more capable of enjoying them. There is more privacy and fewer interruptions, and many couples feel that they have reached a time in their lives where they can proceed more slowly and savor the best moments in sex.

CHANGING SEXUAL RESPONSES

In both sexes, the sexual impulse declines with age but the general pattern differs in men and women. A man's sex drive reaches a peak in the late teens and thereafter gradually diminishes. A woman's sexual feeling reaches a maximum much later in adult life and is sustained on a plateau of responsiveness which, if it is going to decline, tends to decline only in her late 60s. There is much research supporting the existence of a strong sexual urge in 70- and 80-year-old women, just as there is in some men. There is not usually an abrupt loss of sexual feeling and interest coinciding with menopause, as many women fear.

At about the time of menopause, a woman may become anxious about her loss of youthful attractiveness and the fact that any children she might have no longer need her maternal care. These insecurities may make her less ready to respond sexually. At the same time of life, a man usually has reached the most senior position he will attain in his work. If his early ambitions have not been fulfilled, and he feels threatened by younger men, his feelings may find expression in a lack of sexual interest or a feeling of sexual inadequacy. The "male menopause" syndrome is a reality to which many wives will attest. Both men and women may seek escape from this sense of decline by engaging in sexual adventures in a forlorn attempt to recapture the experiences of youth. However, a satisfactory sexual relationship in an older couple is likely to be sustained if the couple enjoys a close understanding, companionship, and mutual respect throughout their middle age. This is entirely within the grasp of most couples, and it is worth planning and working for.

THE EFFECTS OF A LONG-TERM RELATIONSHIP

All-consuming, passionate lovemaking is a rare occurrence. If we set our sights on this romantic ideal and expect it to occur with any frequency, we will almost certainly be disappointed. There are, however, many forms of enjoyable sex and everyone can experience perfectly satisfying sex, which can be quite different on different occasions, with the same partner. This is one of the thrills of a long-term relationship — discovering new ways of enjoying sex by being together over time and gradually making discoveries. For many women an orgasm is not the be-all and end-all of enjoyable sex, and as a man gets older he may not experience an orgasm every time he has sexual intercourse. Many men feel that they have to chase the elusive orgasm with every coital union, but why, when there is so much satisfaction in warm, less passionate sex?

Several pitfalls await us if we continue to believe that sex must be exciting and that only exciting sex is good. This makes us tend to avoid having it unless we are sure that excitement will be an ingredient and, in this way, we narrow the spectrum of attainable experiences and deprive ourselves of peaceful, relaxing, joyful sex. Another unfortunate result is that sex becomes hard work and, as such, is boring and dull.

Hostility, resentment, contempt, and distaste can all ruin a good relationship, even a sound marriage, let alone sexual enjoyment. No good relationship requires an intense, permanent state of rapture or even a permanent emotional commitment. It does, however, require kindness, caring, thoughtfulness, a desire to comfort, and shared intimacy. Problems are bound to arise when one partner has difficulty being warm and close with the other. There may be a steady pulling apart rather than a coming together if one person feels that the other is demanding more affection than he or she feels comfortable about giving. No couple can be close and intimate if there is no basic mutual respect and affection between the partners. In addition to this, no sex therapy can work.

SEX AND THE OLDER MAN

As a man gets older, there is no doubt he experiences a change in the pattern of his sexual activity, and it is important for a man to be open and honest with himself and his partners so that there is enough understanding to sustain a loving relationship.

As a man ages it often takes longer to get an erection or the erection may not last as long as the man would like. Moreover, the erection may not be as full or as hard as before. Many men see such limpness as the beginning of the end.

It may be that a man needs stimulation to maintain an erection. Erection may even refuse to occur for a multitude of reasons, and if it doesn't, a man tends to panic and label himself as impotent. This is the worst thing he can do because the label can create and intensify the problem.

Once a man starts to worry about his erection, he is in a vicious circle because anxiety leads to flaccidity. Insecurity is made worse by the fact that a man who fails to have erections is sometimes labeled impotent. If it is fear or anxiety that is preventing a man from having an erection then it is wrong for him to feel he is impotent. Understandably most men in this situation would feel depressed, but they should certainly not feel like failures.

COPING WITH THE CHANGES There is no grounds for feeling depressed, since impotency due to fear or anxiety can be cured. Masters and Johnson found that any kind of therapy for impotence or premature ejaculation is as successful with older men as it is with younger ones because most of the problems are psychological in origin and have no physical basis whatsoever. The success rate in the older age group is extremely high, so help through counseling or sex therapy should always be sought.

Once a man can relax and stop worrying about his potency, a return to normal sexual activity nearly always follows. It helps if he realizes that it is unnecessary for him to ejaculate every time; rest periods of several days between sexual encounters help both erection and orgasm. If older men respond to their natural rhythms instead of feeling forced by macho instincts to have frequent sex, then their own sex lives come more under their control.

As a man ages it takes him longer to ejaculate. Mastering ejaculatory control is beneficial for both partners, and many men who were particularly quick to ejaculate when younger see this as a gift. Moreover, an older man may not ejaculate every time he has intercourse, and this is also beneficial. Since ejaculation inhibits erection in older men particularly, by not ejaculating at each occasion, he will be able to have more frequent erections.

HELPING AN OLDER MAN

You should make an effort to understand the changes in the way your partner is functioning, and to see each development as perfectly normal. But you may have to change the emphasis of your sexual activity; longer and stronger foreplay, more tactile stimulation including caressing, rubbing, and cuddling, and the use of different sexual positions should be expected.

You must accept the fact that your partner may take longer to attain his erection as he gets older. If you sense apprehension, reassure him and tell him it is fine if he takes longer because it takes you longer, too. An older man, too, may be less aroused by seeing his partner naked than he was before, and as he gets older he needs increasing stimulation in order to achieve erection. This stimulation at some times may be only fantasy, but at other times overt physical stimulation, especially of the penis, is necessary. In these cases, mutual masturbation or oral sex may become more important than it was in earlier years.

Do not panic and do not feel rejected or believe that your partner is no longer attracted to you; do not worry or comment if he does not ejaculate but seems sexually satisfied. In these situations, a woman should see herself as a creator and initiator leading the way and introducing a changing pattern so that both partners create a new kind of sexual loving. In this way, you will help build your partner's self-esteem instead of eroding it.

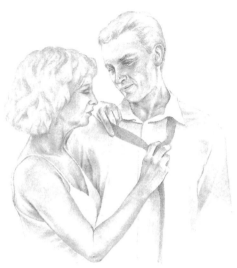

Adapting foreplay
Longer, more prolonged foreplay maybe necessary for arousal — with you taking the lead.

Taking a greater role
Positions that allow you to control the pace take pressure to perform off your partner.

SEX AND THE OLDER WOMAN

Not only do many women write themselves off after they have gone through menopause, but so does society. Society characterizes the older woman as sexless; this is wrong and very cruel. Up until the age of 60, sexual response in women does not change at all. After 60, whatever changes take place are extremely slow and gradual. There are some physiological changes with age, like vaginal lubrication, which from taking only 15 to 30 seconds in the younger woman may take one, two or even five minutes in the older. There may be a thinning and loss of elasticity in the walls of the vagina, plus a shortening of vaginal length and width, changes that have little or no effect on sensation and feeling and orgasm. Eighty percent of older women report no pain or discomfort with intercourse, even though it is a commonly accepted myth that intercourse in an older woman results in discomfort.

Studies show that women have a more stable sex drive than men. Women over 65 continue to seek out, and respond to, erotic encounters, have erotic dreams, and continue to be capable of orgasms, even multiple ones.

Most aspects of arousal remain identical in older women as for younger. Nipples still become erect and the clitoris remains the main organ of sexual stimulation. The excitement generated by clitoral stimulation is exactly the same. A woman of 80 has the same physical potential for orgasm as she did at 20.

CHANGING SEXUAL BEHAVIOR   By far the most important factors influencing the sexual behavior of an older woman are the availability of a partner and the opportunity for regular sexual activity. However, many older women do find themselves without a regular sexual outlet mainly because their partners withdraw from sexual activities from a fear of impotency, or because they have suffered an illness such as a heart attack.

Women reach their sexual peaks later than men, who peak in early adolescence and then show a steady decline throughout life. On the other hand, a woman reaches her peak in her late 20s or 30s, and remains at that plateau until her 60s. So just as many women are reaching and enjoying their sexual maturity, their partner's interest is declining. Now the problem arises: women trying to satisfy their sexual needs without making their mates feel sexually incompetent or impotent.

Masturbation is instrumental in keeping alive an older woman's sexuality and sexual identity, and it will keep her physiological responses in good working order. It is especially important during widowhood, when other sexual release may be limited.

HELPING AN OLDER WOMAN

A man should be especially considerate to his partner during the climacteric years, especially if she fears it and aging. He should tell her of her attractiveness and desirability with compliments and constructive suggestions. Long, leisurely embraces, more attention to foreplay, tender stroking and kissing of the breasts and clitoris are rewarding at any time, but particularly in the older woman.

Longer and stronger foreplay, more tactile stimulation including caressing, rubbing, and cuddling, and the use of different sexual positions should be expected.

The best way to ensure a satisfying, continuing sex life is to have frequent sex. Many women, especially those who have regular intercourse — about once or twice a week — maintain a healthy vaginal condition into advanced old age.

If dryness is a problem, the use of lubricating creams, such as KY Jelly, can be very beneficial. Masturbation increases lubrication and diminishes vaginal pain due to dryness, and few women have difficulty in reaching orgasm through masturbation — so if intercourse does not work, you can help your partner reach a climax through manual or oral stimulation.

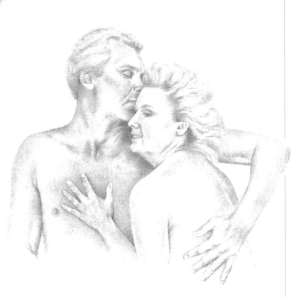

More attention to foreplay
Leisurely embraces and lots of attention to foreplay give an older woman the time she needs to lubricate and prepare for sex.

Use leisure time for leisurely sex
Sensuous massage, stroking her breasts and genitals, keeps a woman feeling attractive and desirable, and more likely to keep wanting to have sex.

KEEPING LOVE ALIVE

Sexual desire in everyone varies from day to day, and like the rest of our behavior, is dependent on what is going on around us. For instance, there is no way that sexual desire can surmount a sudden shock, a severe illness, a bereavement, or an ill child, and it would be foolish to expect it to do so. In fact, the sexual urge is subject to the much smaller ebbs and flows that affect our daily lives, and we should take them in stride and accept them realistically.

Sex may not be enjoyable all the time; just like any other sensory experience, it can be good or bad. While it is realistic and healthy to accept that it can be less than good, having bad sex once does not mean that it will happen frequently or even again for some time. It is a natural variation and should be accepted as such.

Living in close proximity with another person not only reveals our good points but also our negative traits. We all fear in varying degrees that we might not be very lovable and if our partner knew our very worst qualities he or she would not continue to love us, so we have to learn to balance the good with the bad. There is no point in trying to put on a completely fake front; if this does happen in a relationship, tension inevitably builds up and communication begins to deteriorate. If we fail to balance the good with the bad, then we're unable to accept the inevitable criticisms and confrontations that occur as a natural product of life together. Equally, we will feel freer to respond in kind with our own criticisms without feeling a burden of crushing guilt.

MAKING YOUR OWN RULES

There are no universal rules about what people should enjoy in sex or what they shouldn't. As long as couples agree mutually to an activity and neither finds it unpleasant or feels coerced, then there is nothing wrong with enjoying it.

It is perfectly fair to say "No" to your partner if you really do not feel like making love. A good sex life can only be founded on honesty and candor; there is very little to recommend about sex where one partner is faking it. Knowledge of this in retrospect would only make the other partner unhappy.

There are bound to be occasions when one partner wants sex and the other does not, and each has to accept that it is reasonable for that partner to say so, and for sex to be shelved. Of course, in saying no, one has to be entirely honest and say, "No, I want to be left entirely alone," or "I don't feel like sex but I would love to be held."

HAVING
IT
ALL
IN
YOUR
SEX
LIFE

MAKING SEX BETTER

As you learn more about your own sexuality, you will become choosier about your sexual likes and dislikes. As a result, you need to be more ready to discuss them with your partner: sex can have an effect on your overall well-being, and if that effect is negative you have a right to try to improve matters. There is no simple set of rules to follow to guarantee satisfaction. Sexuality is highly individual, and you and your partner should determine what you want out of sex, rather than settle for what others tell you to want.

Not long ago, sexual relationships tended to be dominated by the needs and wants of men, and women didn't complain if their sex lives were unsatisfactory. Today, however, women are more ready to complain because they are better informed and their expectations are higher. Even so, the old attitudes linger on and many women who have sexual problems adopt an attitude of not wanting to make a fuss, instead of doing something about it. That is a mistake, because no-one should underestimate the importance of a satisfactory sex life, or settle for anything less.

SEXUAL INCOMPATIBILITIES

Sexual problems are delicate matters, because they almost always involve someone else at a most intimate level and nobody likes complaints about their sexual behavior. Criticism of someone's sexual performance, no matter how carefully it's worded, can be very hurtful, and men are perhaps more vulnerable to such criticism than women are. Men tend to feel valued for what they do, not for who they are. In their sex lives, they put great emphasis on skills, techniques, timing, and prowess, and this can lead to a high failure rate with anxiety about future success not far below the surface.

Every relationship has its problems from time to time, but with caring on both sides these problems can almost always be resolved by explanation, discussion, and negotiation. Sexual relationships are no exception to this, but dealing with them always requires a great deal of tact and understanding.

If you are unhappy about any aspect of your sex life, think it over carefully before you mention it to your partner. Use the questionnaires on pages 172 to 183 to help you clarify your thoughts about your sexual relationship and to pinpoint any problems or anxieties you might have. Then you can start to discuss the problem with your partner and look for ways to solve it; you'll find some useful guidelines for this on pages 186 to 190. More serious problems that require greater involvement are covered in the next chapter.

MEN'S LIKELY PROBLEM AREAS

Many men treat every sexual encounter as a contest that they will either win or lose. Naturally, they want to win, and according to the common male mythology, that means having a huge penis that becomes instantly erect, stays erect for as long as its owner wants it to, and produces copious amounts of ejaculate.

– DISSATISFACTION WITH GENITALS –

In a recent survey of 1,000 men, almost all of them were very much dissatisfied with the size of their penises, and many felt that they were inadequate. What they didn't realize was that many women couldn't care less about or hardly notice the size of their partner's penis.

Much of a woman's pleasure during intercourse comes from stimulation of her clitoris and of nerve endings situated mainly in the first couple of inches of the vagina, so size really is irrelevant. Apart from that, intercourse is not the only way to enjoy sex. Joy in sexual activities comes in a large part from the stroking, fondling, touching, kissing, licking, nibbling, and hugging that goes on between lovers. Limiting your choices to just getting a hard penis into a vagina as soon as a woman is ready will only add to any performance anxieties you might have.

DISSATISFACTION WITH PERFORMANCE

If you are under the impression that sex should be a spectacular event every time you indulge in it, then sooner or later you are going to be disappointed. There will be times when you can't get properly aroused, and you can't get or sustain an erection or you can't reach an orgasm. There will also be times when you get too aroused, or too anxious about your performance, and you ejaculate prematurely. These things happen to all men from time to time, and you should only think of them as problems if they become persistent.

WOMEN'S LIKELY PROBLEM AREAS

Men, almost without fail, experience an orgasm during sex, and as sex has always been male dominated it was assumed that a woman's experience would be similar. Sadly, this is far from the truth, and the number of women who do not experience an orgasm from intercourse is disappointingly large.

FAKING ORGASM

Many women remain silent about their lack of orgasm, largely to protect their menfolk from embarrassment and loss of face; two out of five married and unmarried women decide that it is less trouble to fake an orgasm than to explain matters to their partners.

Another common reason for a woman to fake orgasm is to avoid being called frigid. The word "frigid" is a destructive label that has no real meaning, but it is too often applied, spitefully, to women who fail to live up to their partners' expectations or who have specific sexual problems. These problems include not being able to have an orgasm, a lack of interest in sex, or experiencing pain or discomfort during intercourse.

– DISAGREEMENT ABOUT ACTIVITIES –

Most usually, the word "frigid" is used to put a woman down for not being as enthusiastic about sex as her partner. In fact, by far the most common point of disagreement between women and their partners is over how often they should have sex. About half of all women feel that their opinion about this differs from that of their partners; most of the time the women want less sex than the men.

It is a woman's right not to feel like having sex sometimes without having to fear being labeled frigid. In any case, most sex therapists believe that frigidity doesn't exist, that all "frigidity" is treatable and that dislike of sex can be overcome.

IS THERE A PROBLEM?

If you have a sexual problem, you will not be able to tackle it unless you first identify it and then examine it carefully. To find out if you actually do have a problem, fill out one of the questionnaires below. Then get your partner to fill in his or her

MAN'S QUESTIONNAIRE

1 Do you think there is something lacking in your sex life?

2 Do you want to change your sex life?

3 Is your partner dissatisfied with you as a sexual partner?

4 Does anxiety interfere with your sexual activities?

5 Are you ashamed or uncomfortable about some part of your body?

6 Do you feel that you're too hard on yourself and that you really aren't as bad as you sometimes make yourself out to be?

7 Are there forms of sexual activity that you would like to engage in that you don't at present?

8 Do you have some problem areas in your feelings about love and sex?

9 Do your sexual fantasies, either while having sex or at other times, interfere with your sexual relationship?

10 Do you have any fears related to sex?

11 Do you feel that you give your partner more pleasure during sex than she gives you?

12 Do you feel guilty about any of your sexual activities?

13 Are you bored with your sexual activities?

14 Do you find sex, or aspects of it, distasteful?

15 Do you have problems on those occasions when you want to tell your partner that you don't want sex?

16 Do you have problems on those occasions when your partner tells you that she doesn't want sex?

17 Are you currently experiencing problems in other aspects of your life that may affect your sex life?

18 Do you and your partner have an unequal interest in sex?

19 Do your preferred sexual activities differ from those of your partner?

20 Do you feel that you are "abnormal" in terms of your sexual interests ?

21 Do you feel that your partner is "abnormal" in terms of her sexual interests or activities?

22 Do you have any physical illnesses, or are you taking any medication, that may affect your sexual responses?

answers to the questions on the appropriate questionnaire. A "yes" answer
to any of the questions will highlight a possible problem area; this usually
can be solved by open discussions between you and your partner.

YES ☐
NO ☐

WOMAN'S QUESTIONNAIRE

1 Do you think there is something lacking in your sex life? ☐ ☐

2 Do you want to change your sex life? ☐ ☐

3 Is your partner dissatisfied with you as a sexual partner? ☐ ☐

4 Does anxiety interfere with your sexual activities? ☐ ☐

5 Are you ashamed or uncomfortable about some part of your body? ☐ ☐

6 Do you feel that you're too hard on yourself and that you really aren't as bad as you sometimes make yourself out to be? ☐ ☐

7 Are there forms of sexual activity that you would like to engage in that you don't at present? ☐ ☐

8 Do you have some problem areas in your feelings about love and sex? ☐ ☐

9 Do your sexual fantasies, either while having sex or at other times, interfere with your sexual relationship? ☐ ☐

10 Do you have any fears related to sex? ☐ ☐

11 Do you feel that you give your partner more pleasure during sex than he gives you? ☐ ☐

12 Do you feel guilty about any of your sexual activities? ☐ ☐

13 Are you bored with your sexual activities? ☐ ☐

14 Do you find sex, or aspects of it, distasteful? ☐ ☐

15 Do you have problems on those occasions when you want to tell your partner that you don't want sex? ☐ ☐

16 Do you have problems on those occasions when your partner tells you that he doesn't want sex? ☐ ☐

17 Are you currently experiencing problems in other aspects of your life that may affect your sex life? ☐ ☐

18 Do you and your partner have an unequal interest in sex? ☐ ☐

19 Do your preferred sexual activities differ from those of your partner? ☐ ☐

20 Do you feel that you are "abnormal" in terms of your sexual interests? ☐ ☐

21 Do you feel that your partner is "abnormal" in terms of his sexual interests or activities? ☐ ☐

22 Do you have any physical illnesses, or are you taking any medication, that may affect your sexual responses? ☐ ☐

WHAT IS MY SEX LIFE LIKE?

As a first step toward solving your sexual problems, it will help if you examine your actual sexual behavior. These questionnaires will give you and your partner a clear picture of what each of you does and doesn't do. Both of you should fill in your individual questionnaires. Use the following letter code to rate the frequency of the

MAN'S QUESTIONNAIRE

1 You talk warmly or sexily to your partner ☐

Your partner talks warmly or sexily to you ☐

2 You stroke your partner's clothed body ☐

Your partner strokes your clothed body ☐

3 You hold or rub yourself against your partner's body ☐

Your partner holds or rubs herself against your body ☐

4 You kiss your partner ☐

Your partner kisses you ☐

5 You undress your partner and look at her nude body ☐

Your partner undresses you and looks at your nude body ☐

6 You stroke your partner's body, including her breasts ☐

Your partner strokes your body ☐

7 You stroke your partner's vagina and clitoris ☐

Your partner stimulates your penis by hand ☐

8 You lick and suck your partner's body, including her breasts ☐

Your partner licks and sucks your body, including your nipples ☐

9 You stimulate your penis by hand ☐

Your partner masturbates in front of you ☐

10 You use your hands on your partner's vagina and clitoris to bring her to orgasm ☐

Your partner uses her hands on your penis to bring you to orgasm ☐

11 You have intercourse to orgasm in the following positions:

You on top ☐

Your partner on top ☐

Side-by-side ☐

You behind your partner ☐

Sitting ☐

Kneeling ☐

Standing ☐

12 You lick or suck in and around your partner's vagina and bring her to orgasm using your mouth ☐

Your partner licks or sucks your penis to bring you to orgasm ☐

13 You caress or kiss your partner's buttocks or anus ☐

Your partner caresses or kisses your buttocks or anus ☐

Never $\boxed{\text{N}}$
Rarely $\boxed{\text{R}}$
Often $\boxed{\text{O}}$
Usually $\boxed{\text{U}}$
Every time $\boxed{\text{E}}$

various activities: N – it never occurs; R – it occurs rarely (less than 25% of the time); O – it occurs fairly often (about 50% of the time); U – it occurs usually (about 75% of the time); E – it occurs every time (100% of the time). Afterward, compare and discuss the results with your partner.

WOMAN'S QUESTIONNAIRE

1 You talk warmly or sexily to your partner ☐

Your partner talks warmly or sexily to you ☐

2 You stroke your partner's clothed body ☐

Your partner strokes your clothed body ☐

3 You hold or rub yourself against your partner's body ☐

Your partner holds or rubs himself against your body ☐

4 You kiss your partner ☐

Your partner kisses you ☐

5 You undress your partner and look at his nude body ☐

Your partner undresses you and looks at your nude body ☐

6 You stroke your partner's body ☐

Your partner strokes your body, including your breasts ☐

7 You stimulate your partner's penis by hand ☐

Your partner strokes your vagina and clitoris ☐

8 You lick and suck your partner's body, including his nipples ☐

Your partner licks and sucks your body, including your breasts ☐

9 You use your hands on your partner's penis to bring him to orgasm ☐

Your partner uses his hands on your vagina and clitoris to bring you to orgasm ☐

10 You have intercourse to orgasm in the following positions:

You on top ☐

Your partner on top ☐

Side-by-side ☐

Your partner behind you ☐

Sitting ☐

Kneeling ☐

Standing ☐

11 You lick or suck your partner's penis to bring him to orgasm ☐

Your partner licks or sucks your vagina and clitoris to bring you to orgasm ☐

12 You caress or kiss your partner's buttocks or anus ☐

Your partner caresses or kisses your buttocks or anus ☐

WHAT SHOULD MY SEX LIFE BE LIKE?

Now that you and your partner have discussed what actually happens within your sexual relationship, the next step is to think about what each of you would like to happen. These questionnaires will enable both of you to learn more about the other's sexual preferences, and show you what each can do to increase the other's enjoyment of sex. As before, you and your partner should fill them in separately with your rat-

MAN'S QUESTIONNAIRE

1 You talk warmly or sexily to your partner ☐

Your partner talks warmly or sexily to you ☐

2 You stroke your partner's clothed body ☐

Your partner strokes your clothed body ☐

3 You hold or rub yourself against your partner's body ☐

Your partner holds or rubs herself against your body ☐

4 You kiss your partner ☐

Your partner kisses you ☐

5 You undress your partner and look at her nude body ☐

Your partner undresses you and looks at your nude body ☐

6 You stroke your partner's body, including her breasts ☐

Your partner strokes your body ☐

7 You stroke your partner's vagina and clitoris ☐

8 You lick and suck your partner's body, including her breasts ☐

Your partner licks and sucks your body, including your nipples ☐

9 You stimulate your penis by hand ☐

Your partner stimulates your penis by hand ☐

10 You use your hands on your partner's clitoris to bring her to orgasm ☐

Your partner uses her hands on your penis to bring you to orgasm ☐

11 You have intercourse to orgasm in the following positions:

You on top ☐

Your partner on top ☐

Side-by-side ☐

You behind your partner ☐

Sitting ☐

Kneeling ☐

Standing ☐

12 You bring your partner to orgasm using your mouth ☐

Your partner licks or sucks your penis to bring you to orgasm ☐

13 You caress or kiss your partner's buttocks or anus ☐

Your partner caresses or kisses your buttocks or anus ☐

Never	N
Rarely	R
Often	O
Usually	U
Every time	E

ings: N – wish it never occurred; R – would like it rarely (no more than 25% of the time); O – would like it fairly often (about 50% of the time); U – would like it to occur usually (about 75% of the time); E – would like it every time (100% of the time). Afterward, discuss and compare your ratings together.

WOMAN'S QUESTIONNAIRE

1 You talk warmly or sexily to your partner ☐

Your partner talks warmly or sexily to you ☐

2 You stroke your partner's clothed body ☐

Your partner strokes your clothed body ☐

3 You hold or rub yourself against your partner's body ☐

Your partner holds or rubs himself against your body ☐

4 You kiss your partner ☐

Your partner kisses you ☐

5 You undress your partner and look at his nude body ☐

Your partner undresses you and looks at your nude body ☐

6 You stroke your partner's body ☐

Your partner strokes your body, including your breasts ☐

7 Your partner strokes your vagina and clitoris ☐

8 You stimulate your partner's penis by hand ☐

9 You lick and suck your partner's body, including his nipples ☐

Your partner licks and sucks your body, including your nipples ☐

10 You use your hands on your partner's penis to bring him to orgasm ☐

Your partner uses his hands on your vagina and clitoris to bring you to orgasm ☐

11 You have intercourse to orgasm in the following positions:

You on top ☐

Your partner on top ☐

Side-by-side ☐

Your partner behind you ☐

Sitting ☐

Kneeling ☐

Standing ☐

12 You lick or suck your partner's penis to bring him to orgasm ☐

Your partner licks or sucks your vagina and clitoris to bring you to orgasm ☐

13 You caress or kiss your partner's buttocks or anus ☐

Your partner caresses or kisses your buttocks or anus ☐

HOW DO I FEEL ABOUT MY PARTNER?

As with all relationships, you're bound to have some fairly strong feelings about your partner, and these certainly will affect your sexual behavior and satisfaction. One way of getting your feelings out in the open is to answer the following questions.

MAN'S QUESTIONNAIRE

1 Was your first sexual experience with your partner a success? If not, why not?

. . . .

. . . .

2 Have your sexual feelings toward her changed? If so, how?

. . . .

. . . .

3 Is there something you especially like about your sexual experiences with her? If there is, what is it?

. . . .

. . . .

4 Is there something you especially dislike about your sexual experiences with her? If there is, what is it?

. . . .

. . . .

5 Is there something you would like to change in your sexual contacts with your partner? If there is, what is it?

. . . .

. . . .

6 Is there anything you would like your partner to do when you make love that she doesn't do now? If so, what is it?

. . . .

. . . .

7 Is there anything your partner does when you make love that you wish she wouldn't do? If there is, what is it?

. . . .

. . . .

8 Do you feel comfortable about discussing your sexual behavior and attitudes with your partner? If not, why not?

. . . .

. . . .

9 Do you encounter any problems when you try to have an open, positive discussion about sex with your partner? If you do, what are they?

. . . .

. . . .

10 Are there any problems with your relationship as a whole that you feel interfere with your sexual relationship? If so, what are they?

. . . .

. . . .

11 Do you share outside interests and friendships with your partner?

. . . .

. . . .

. . . .

Each of you should fill in your appropriate questionnaire, checking the "yes" or "no" box as appropriate, and adding any relevant information that you can. When you have finished, discuss each other's answers in the spirit of implementing some changes.

YES ☐

NO ☐

WOMAN'S QUESTIONNAIRE

1 Was your first sexual experience with your partner a success? If not, why not? ☐ ☐

. . . .

. . . .

2 Have your sexual feelings toward him changed? If so, how? ☐ ☐

. . . .

. . . .

3 Is there something you especially like about your sexual experiences with him? If there is, what is it? ☐ ☐

. . . .

. . . .

4 Is there something you especially dislike about your sexual experiences with him? If there is, what is it? ☐ ☐

. . . .

. . . .

5 Is there something you would like to change in your sexual contacts with your partner? If there is, what is it? ☐ ☐

. . . .

. . . .

6 Is there anything you would like your partner to do when you make love that he doesn't do now? If so, what is it? ☐ ☐

. . . .

. . . .

7 Is there anything your partner does when you make love that you wish he wouldn't do? If there is, what is it? ☐ ☐

. . . .

. . . .

8 Do you feel comfortable about discussing your sexual behavior and attitudes with your partner? If not, why not? ☐ ☐

. . . .

. . . .

9 Do you encounter problems when you try to have an open, positive discussion about sex with him? If you do, what are they? ☐ ☐

. . . .

. . . .

10 Are there any problems with your relationship as a whole that you feel interfere with your sexual relationship? If so, what are they? ☐ ☐

. . . .

. . . .

11 Do you share outside interests and friendships with your partner? ☐ ☐

. . . .

. . . .

. . . .

MAN: WHAT AM I ANXIOUS ABOUT?

For a man, the most common obstacle to enjoying sex is a feeling of anxiety, arising from feelings of guilt, embarrassment, or inhibition, or from fear of not being able to perform adequately. Tension caused by anxiety will seriously interfere with your sexual pleasure and may prevent you from becoming aroused, getting or maintaining an erection, reaching orgasm, or it may cause you to ejaculate prematurely. If you have anxieties, you may not know exactly what they are about, so here are some questions that will help you to pinpoint their causes.

1 Do sexual activities in general make you anxious?

. . . .

. . . .

2 Are there certain situations in which sex makes you feel uncomfortable — for example, with a particular partner, in a particular place or at a particular time? Please specify.

. . . .

. . . .

3 Do any of the following create particular anxiety for you?

Not getting erect

Getting turned on when your partner doesn't

Stimulating yourself when you're alone

Stimulating yourself when you're with your partner

Oral sex

Anal sex

Certain positions in intercourse (if so, which?)

. . . .

. . . .

Wanting certain things from your partner but being shy about asking for them (if so, which things?)

. . . .

. . . .

Being asked for certain things by your partner (if so, which things?) Anything else?

. . . .

. . . .

4 Which sexual activities or situations make you feel most relaxed?

. . . .

. . . .

5 Are there any particular sexual fantasies that make you feel anxious? If there are, what are they?

. . . .

. . . .

When you have answered the questions, read your "yes" answers again and think about what they reveal about your sexual anxieties. Can you pinpoint when anxieties occur and under what conditions? Is there any way you can avoid those situations that make you anxious or, better yet, is there any way you can reduce the amount of anxiety they cause you? Perhaps your partner can give you some ideas. It's also possible that talking over those things may help to reduce your anxiety.

YES ☐
NO ☐

6 Do you have a fear of failure in sex or concerns about disappointing your partner? ☐ ☐

. . . .

. . . .

7 Can you think of any past experiences concerning sex that could be connected with present anxieties? If you can, what are they? ☐ ☐

. . . .

. . . .

8 What is there, if anything, about yourself that makes you anxious about sex (for example, the size, shape or appearance of your penis)?

. . . .

. . . .

9 Complete the following sentences relating to your sexual activities as fast as you can with the words or phrases that first occur to you:

I wish I could . . . .

. . . .

I love it when . . . .

. . . .

I'm afraid to . . . .

. . . .

I get scared when . . . .

. . . .

I'm afraid I will . . . .

. . . .

I get uncomfortable when my partner . .

. . . .

I get uncomfortable when I . . . .

. . . .

I get embarrassed when I . . . .

. . . .

I get embarrassed when my partner . . . .

. . . .

I wish I didn't . . . .

. . . .

I wish my partner would . . . .

. . . .

I wish my partner wouldn't . . . .

. . . .

I'd love to be able to . . . .

. . . .

I'm afraid I won't . . . .

. . . .

I'm terrified of . . . .

. . . .

WOMAN: WHAT AM I ANXIOUS ABOUT?

For a woman, the most common obstacle to enjoying sex is a feeling of anxiety, arising from feelings of inhibition, embarrassment, or guilt, or from fear of not being able to be sexually satisfying for a partner. Tension caused by anxiety will seriously interfere with a woman's sexual pleasure, and may prevent you from becoming aroused, excited, or reaching orgasm. If you have anxieties concerning sex, you may not know exactly what they are about, so here are some questions that will help you to pinpoint their causes.

1 Do sexual activities in general make you anxious?

. . . .

. . . .

2 Are there certain situations in which sex makes you feel uncomfortable — for example, with a particular partner, in a particular place, or at a particular time? Please specify.

. . . .

. . . .

3 Do any of the following create particular anxiety for you?

Not getting aroused (not lubricating)

Getting turned on when your partner doesn't

Stimulating yourself when you're alone

Stimulating yourself when you're with your partner

Oral sex

Anal sex

Certain positions in intercourse (if so, which?)

. . . .

. . . .

Wanting certain things from your partner but being shy about asking for them (if so, which things?)

. . . .

. . . .

Being asked for certain things by your partner (if so, which things?) Anything else?

. . . .

. . . .

4 Which sexual activities or situations make you feel most relaxed?

. . . .

. . . .

5 Are there any particular sexual fantasies that make you feel anxious? If there are, what are they?

. . . .

. . . .

. . . .

When you have answered them, read your "yes" answers again and think about what they tell about your sexual anxieties. Can you pinpoint when they occur and under what conditions? Is there any way you can avoid those situations that make you anxious or, better yet, is there any way you can reduce the amount of anxiety they cause you? Perhaps your partner can give you some ideas. It's also possible that talking over these things may help to reduce your anxiety.

YES ☐
NO ☐

6   Do you have a fear of failure in sex or concerns about disappointing your partner? ☐ ☐

. . . .

. . . .

7   Can you think of any past experiences concerning sex that could be connected with present anxieties? If you can, what are they? ☐ ☐

. . . .

. . . .

8   What is there, if anything, about yourself that makes you anxious about sex (for example, the way you behave when you get turned on)?

. . . .

. . . .

9   Complete the following sentences relating to your sexual activities as fast as you can with the words or phrases that first occur to you:

I wish I could . . . .

. . . .

I love it when . . . .

. . . .

I'm afraid to . . . .

. . . .

I get scared when . . . .

. . . .

I'm afraid I will . . . .

. . . .

I get uncomfortable when my partner . .

. . . .

I get uncomfortable when I . . . .

. . . .

I get embarrassed when I . . . .

. . . .

I get embarrassed when my partner . . . .

. . . .

I wish I didn't . . . .

. . . .

I wish my partner would . . . .

. . . .

I wish my partner wouldn't . . . .

. . . .

I'd love to be able to . . . .

. . . .

I'm afraid I won't . . . .

. . . .

I'm terrified of . . . .

. . . .

EXPRESSING WHAT YOU WANT

Frequently, an obstacle to full sexual enjoyment arises when partners don't explain their needs and their likes and dislikes to each other. There are many reasons for this, such as embarrassment or a reluctance to discuss sex because of social, moral, or religious attitudes. More often, though, it's because one or both partners in a relationship has no clear idea of what, for them, makes sex enjoyable.

If you want a truly fulfilling sex life, it's essential that you establish what conditions will allow you to have sex in the way you want it. You owe this to yourself, and to your partner, and you have the right to do it. By communicating fully and openly, you should try to come as close to the conditions you prefer as you can both negotiate.

WHAT IS IT YOU WANT?

As a first step, think back to those sexual experiences that you have enjoyed most and try to work out what it was that made each of them so enjoyable. What was there about them that most turned you on? Who was your partner, where were you, and what was the situation? What did you and your partner do with each other, and what aspects of the encounter do you remember most vividly?

Next, think about those sexual encounters that didn't turn out so well (if you're one of those rare people who have never had a dud sexual experience, try to imagine some really bad ones). Who were you with and how did you feel about him or her? Where were you, what were the circumstances, and what exactly did you do? What was there about those encounters that made them less than pleasant?

Now compare your best experiences with your worst ones, and make a list of any significant factors that you think make sex good for you, and a list of those that you think make it bad. Your lists will probably include items about your feelings toward your partner, and your ability to turn your partner on and to get really turned on yourself. Other items might touch on such factors as whether you were able to focus on your lovemaking and forget about everything else, the quality and comfort of the surroundings, your anxiety (or lack of it), and fears about performance, pregnancy, or disease.

Make the items on your lists as specific as possible. Then rewrite the lists, placing the most important items at the top and the least important at the bottom. These revised lists will show you what, for you, are the conditions you need for good sex, and the conditions you want to avoid because they can lead to bad sex.

Finally, think about the items on your lists. Do you think they are reasonable, and how do they apply to your relationship with your present partner? Do you think you can work with your partner to achieve more of the "good" conditions, if any are missing from your relationship, and to eliminate any of the "bad" ones that may exist?

EXPRESSING YOUR NEEDS

At one time or another, you have probably expected your partner to be a mind reader or to be able to tell instinctively what you did or did not want. That is expecting far too much: your partner can only respond to your sexual predilections if you tell him or her what they are.

So stating your needs is important, but choose carefully when and how you do so. The time to talk about your sexual preferences is when both you and your partner are feeling warm, close, and intimate. There are many times when you should not raise the subject — especially when you or your partner feel angry, frustrated, cheated, or resentful. You should also avoid the subject when you are feeling vulnerable to criticism or when your feelings are hurt, because then you may start to use sex as a lever to manipulate your partner. If you do this, your relationship could start to go downhill fast.

If you choose the time and your words carefully, there will be little risk of offending your partner by discussing your sexual needs. But if your words are hostile, offensive, barbed, or full of accusations, you will hurt your partner and probably end up having a fight and damaging your relationship. Sexual criticism cuts deep, and is not easily forgotten.

The best way to approach the subject is to begin by talking about the good points of your sex life and giving praise where it is due. Then you can gently lead the conversation around to the changes you would like to make, perhaps by mentioning something you would like to do more often, or for longer, or in a different way. Once you're safely on the subject of change, you might want to suggest doing something you would like that you haven't done before, or not doing something that you haven't been enjoying.

Always keep your comments and suggestions positive, and above all remember that you are having a discussion with your partner, not presenting a list of demands. Your partner may well have his or her own suggestions for change, and you should respond to these with the same sensitivity as you expect your own ideas to receive.

At the end of one of these conversations it could turn out that you both have many good points to emphasize and to work on together. But if not many positive feelings and suggestions have come to light, you will need to agree on some kind of plan of action, such as the one on the next page, to improve your sexual relations.

PLANNING FOR CHANGE

If your conversations with your partner have revealed many flaws in your sexual relationship, you will need to work together to overcome your difficulties. It can be hard to know where to start, and if that is the case it helps to have a definite plan to follow, such as the one described here, which leads you through a series of short discussions. It has a simple structure that allows each of you to state your point of view and to respond to what the other is saying, so as to keep the discussions fair and balanced.

Set aside approximately half an hour, no more than once a day, for each discussion. Neither of you should try to coerce the other into going beyond the half hour, but you can continue longer if you both want to. The diagram opposite shows you how to organize each session, and below are some suggested topics for you to talk about.

THE FIRST SESSIONS

In your first session you should concentrate on describing how you feel about the good parts of your relationship. It's important to recognize the positive aspects so you can preserve and build on them.

After the first session, take a few minutes to discuss it and to agree on any changes to the "rules" you might want to make for future sessions. It's important that you do this so that you establish a procedure that you are both happy with. You should also discuss how comfortable you each feel about talking over your sexual relationship, and any problems you think you might have in communicating your feelings and wishes in subsequent sessions.

In your second session, you should each try to suggest ways in which you can improve your own behavior in bed. Can you recognize any needs of your partner that are not being met? What more do you feel you can give your partner?

The first two sessions should be relatively straightforward, and will give you a positive basis for your future discussions. In these, you can really get down to examining what is wrong and looking for ways to solve your problems. During the course of these sessions, each of you should consider the following questions:

- What would you like from your partner that you are not getting or not getting enough of?
- Are there things you wish your partner would do more often, for longer, or differently?
- Are there things you wish your partner would not do, or do less often?

- Are there positions for intercourse or other forms of stimulation that you would like to use more often?
- Are there any problems with the timing of when you make love, the events that lead up to it, or what happens after it?

– TALKING THROUGH YOUR PROBLEMS –

While it may seem strange at first to discuss your problems formally, it is often the only way that anything can be resolved. Partners must take turns speaking and having the full attention of their listener.

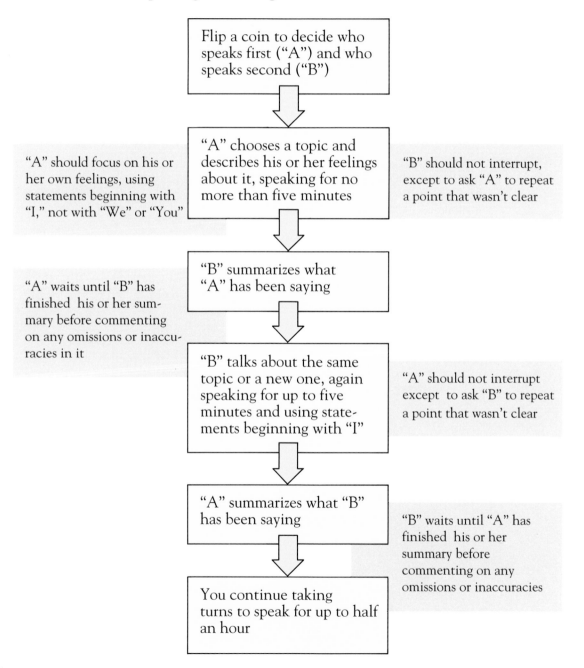

Flip a coin to decide who speaks first ("A") and who speaks second ("B")

"A" should focus on his or her own feelings, using statements beginning with "I," not with "We" or "You"

"A" chooses a topic and describes his or her feelings about it, speaking for no more than five minutes

"B" should not interrupt, except to ask "A" to repeat a point that wasn't clear

"A" waits until "B" has finished his or her summary before commenting on any omissions or inaccuracies in it

"B" summarizes what "A" has been saying

"B" talks about the same topic or a new one, again speaking for up to five minutes and using statements beginning with "I"

"A" should not interrupt except to ask "B" to repeat a point that wasn't clear

"A" summarizes what "B" has been saying

"B" waits until "A" has finished his or her summary before commenting on any omissions or inaccuracies

You continue taking turns to speak for up to half an hour

— Making The Correct Responses —

Listen carefully to your partner's ideas and respond to them sensitively, explaining how you feel about his or her requests. Are they news to you? How reasonable do you think they are? Can you handle them? Think carefully about each point before you reply to it, and remember that in giving your partner what he or she wants, you are going to be getting something back in return because your mutual joy will be enhanced.

However, it might happen that one of you is making requests that the other cannot agree to, at least at this time. If so, you will need to negotiate a compromise, remembering that negotiations involve give and take, not making demands and sticking to them regardless of what your partner feels.

Once you have agreed on the changes you want to make, you can start thinking about how and when you want to introduce them. You can, of course, do this right away, but if you prefer to do it gradually you might find that drawing up some form of schedule will help you to plan ahead. This schedule should meet the needs of both you and your partner, and you should both be in agreement about what you will do, and how often and when.

—— Helps In Achieving Success ——

If you want a written agreement, try putting it in the form of a contract. A contract does help when you have a problem to solve or a goal to reach, and it ensures that both of you agree and understand what you are going to do. Opposite is the sort of contract that you might use; it sets out goals, rewards, timing, and so forth.

If this contract is a success, you might want to go on to draw up a similar one for a program of arousal and erotic pleasure exercises. These are the sensate focus exercises that help you relax and stimulate all your senses and enhance your sexuality (see pages 198 to 201). They make you focus on activities other than genital sex, so that you come to understand that there are many other forms of sex than sexual intercourse. In the first of the exercises, genital contact is excluded; you then go on to manual and oral-genital contact, but without sexual intercourse. That will come later, and you might want to make it the subject of another contract.

By using a report form of some sort, such as the one on page 190, you can record your enjoyment and success with the exercises. It will give you a clear picture of how you are progressing, and show you if you should stay with a particular exercise for a while – until you are successful at it – before moving on to the next. You can, of course, modify your contracts or report forms to suit your own circumstances.

CONTRACT

We, the undersigned, will attempt to improve our sexual relationship in a particular way by working through a series of mutually agreed-upon steps and rewards for a certain period of time.

ULTIMATE GOAL

. . . .
. . . .

SPECIFIC STEPS

STEP	GOAL FOR STEP
1	1 . . . .
. . . .	. . . .
2	2 . . . .
. . . .	. . . .
3	3 . . . .
. . . .	. . . .
4	4 . . . .
. . . .	. . . .

Number of Sessions: . . . .   Location of Sessions . . . .
. . . .

What you will do for your partner   . . . .
. . . .

What your partner will do for you   . . . .
. . . .

REWARDS

After each session   . . . .
After completion of each step   . . . .
At the end of each week   . . . .

Other details (for example, how you will compromise or renegotiate the contract, or what you will do if one of you can't fulfill the contract):

. . . .
. . . .

AGREED AND SIGNED

Date   Date

. . . .

REPORT FORM

DAY	EXERCISE AGREED UPON	EXERCISE COMPLETED		DEGREE OF SUCCESS			REWARD GIVEN	
		YES	NO	NONE	PARTIAL	COMPLETE	YES	NO

SUCCESS
WITH
YOUR
SEXUAL
PROBLEMS

SEXUAL PROBLEMS

In a long-term relationship, it is a rare couple who won't experience some problem with their sex life. And when it occurs, it always will involve both partners. It was Masters and Johnson who first said that there is no such thing as an uninvolved partner in a sexual problem. If you have a sexual problem, there is no way in which your partner will not be involved, whether it is his or her sexual fulfillment being limited by your problem, or his or her having a role in developing and maintaining your problem in the first place.

And that is another reason why communciation within couples is so important. Without open and frank discussions, a serious problem won't ever be solved, and a less serious one can magnify. Unfortunately, however, some couples have unspoken contracts that prevent them from talking about their sexual problems and inadequacies, because they fear doing so will create a threat to the balance of their relationship. Yet it is no relationship when one or both partners is not experiencing a happy sexual relationship and whose chance of salvaging it is blocked.

— THE MOST COMMON COMPLAINTS —

Contrary to what most people believe, the sexual problems usually encountered by couples are not normally due to physical problems but to the following:

- Fear of sex
- Discomfort with intimacy
- Pressure to be a sexual athlete
- Lack of sexual knowledge
- Lack of effective communication
- Lack of consensus on sexual activity
- Problems with boring and distasteful sex

And it's just this sort of problem that can best be solved within a couple by an open attitude to sex and communication. There are, however, some conditions with physiological implications that make intercourse difficult as well as painful, and the management of these is covered below.

For women, lack of orgasm and unresponsiveness make love-making a less than rewarding, though a still possible, experience, while pain during intercourse makes it unbearable. For men, problems with ejaculation makes sex less good for both partners, while erection difficulties can make it impossible. Both partners can suffer emotional problems that can be destructive not only to their entire relationship but to their sex life in particular. It is vital that all problems, once identified, be treated as soon as possible and with professional help, if necessary.

WOMEN'S PROBLEMS

Except for painful sex, which can have psychological as well as physiological causes, a woman's sex problems do not normally prevent her from engaging in intercourse — another major difference between the sexes. They do, however, impair her enjoyment of sex, and lead to a disinclination to continue having it. Without being responsive to sexual feeling or experiencing orgasms as desired, a woman will never be an equal sexual partner.

UNRESPONSIVENESS

Usually a woman who is unresponsive feels little need to be satisfied by the man with whom she is making love. She tends to submit to sex without really wanting it; she may even feel that sex is something that she has to bear. It corresponds very closely to the old idea that women should remain passive so that a man can take his pleasure. This may sound ridiculous taken in the context of today's liberated woman, but many women still cling to this outdated notion. As the woman feels unable to take part in the proceedings, arousal is minimal, and there will be little physical warmth in her lovemaking. Mentally, a woman will hold back, and physically, she will be very inhibited.

There may be many reasons for a woman feeling like this: she may have had a disturbing sexual encounter when she was young; she may have been brought up to think that sex is dirty; she may never have been awoken erotically before, and simply does not know how to respond to sexual sensations in her body. Her man could be selfish, in a hurry, lacking in technique, or unsympathetic to female sexuality. Both partners may be immature and full of false illusions about sex. Whenever a man meets such a situation, he should stop and try to discuss matters sympathetically with his partner; no woman is truly frigid. With sympathetic help from a partner, or with sex counseling, apparent frigidity can always be remedied.

Where unresponsiveness is a problem, partners should guarantee themselves enough time and privacy for sex so that you shouldn't feel rushed or worry about interruptions; you should also avoid discussing major worries prior to sex, and should resolve any quarrels long before bedtime.

If either partner is feeling tense or anxious, you can practice relaxation exercises or have a glass of wine to calm down. The woman should concentrate on her feelings, and not be made to worry or feel rushed about achieving orgasm. It is important, too, that sufficient foreplay is indulged in so that a woman is fully aroused. The sensate focus exercises on pages 198 to 201 should be explored.

UNRESPONSIVENESS

THE MAN'S EXPERIENCE This man's partner appears to have no desire to make love to him at all. She seems to bear his making love to her as if it is an unpleasant duty. He tries to stimulate her in different ways, but she doesn't respond. When they make love, he reaches an orgasm — but without any response from her it feels more like a biological function than an act of passion. He is beginning to feel that he is an inadequate lover and the sexual part of their relationship is becoming a barrier; he is even beginning to resent her for making him feel perverted because he wants to make love.

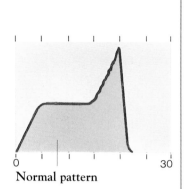

Normal pattern

ORGASM

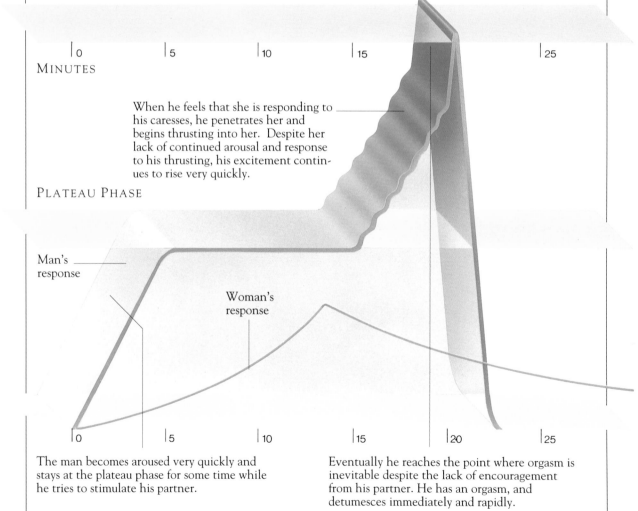

MINUTES

| 0 | 5 | 10 | 15 | 25 |

When he feels that she is responding to his caresses, he penetrates her and begins thrusting into her. Despite her lack of continued arousal and response to his thrusting, his excitement continues to rise very quickly.

PLATEAU PHASE

Man's response

Woman's response

The man becomes aroused very quickly and stays at the plateau phase for some time while he tries to stimulate his partner.

Eventually he reaches the point where orgasm is inevitable despite the lack of encouragement from his partner. He has an orgasm, and detumesces immediately and rapidly.

THE WOMAN'S EXPERIENCE This woman does not feel the need to have much physical contact with her present partner, and certainly would never initiate sex because she feels that it is unnatural for a woman to demand sex from a man. She tries to divorce herself from the act when she occasionally submits, feeling that if she responds she is in some way dirty. Sometimes she feels mild sexual excitement, but this soon dies away as her feelings of guilt overcome it. She puts up with having sex only because it seems to be important to her partner.

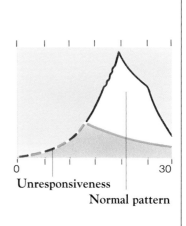

0   30
Unresponsiveness
Normal pattern

ORGASM

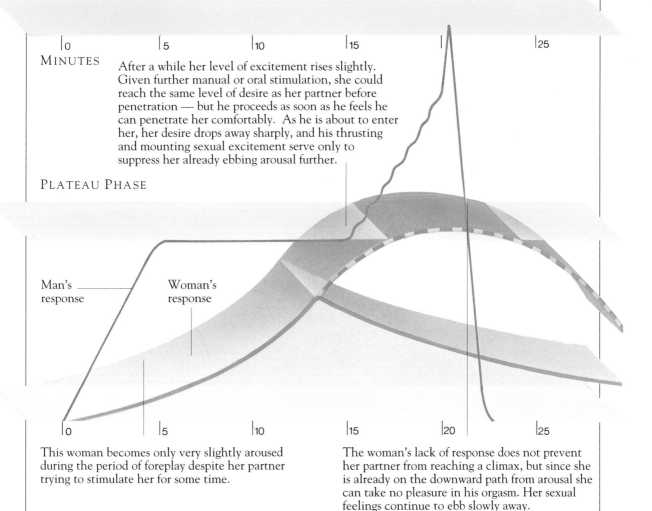

MINUTES

0   5   10   15   25

After a while her level of excitement rises slightly. Given further manual or oral stimulation, she could reach the same level of desire as her partner before penetration — but he proceeds as soon as he feels he can penetrate her comfortably. As he is about to enter her, her desire drops away sharply, and his thrusting and mounting sexual excitement serve only to suppress her already ebbing arousal further.

PLATEAU PHASE

Man's response

Woman's response

0   5   10   15   20   25

This woman becomes only very slightly aroused during the period of foreplay despite her partner trying to stimulate her for some time.

The woman's lack of response does not prevent her partner from reaching a climax, but since she is already on the downward path from arousal she can take no pleasure in his orgasm. Her sexual feelings continue to ebb slowly away.

SENSATE FOCUS

When a person has been sexually unresponsive for some time, it is important to reawaken the sexual feelings gradually, and to relearn how to give and receive pleasure. Most sex therapists, in treating unresponsiveness, use a form of sensual massage that allows a person to explore his or her own body and that of their partner. This sensate focusing enables couples to give and receive pleasure through touch alone, with the mutual agreement that sexual intercourse is delayed for some time. During these exercises it is important to focus on the pleasurable sensations you are feeling now, at the current moment, instead of anticipating or worrying about intercourse. Intercourse and orgasm are not the usual goals, though if these "exercises" are successful, it will almost certainly stimulate your appetite for intercourse.

Alternate between
the front and back
of your hand

Concentrate on yourself
Be sure to pick a time and a place where you won't be disturbed. Start by touching yourself all over, trying to focus your senses on what feels good, and what arouses you. Stroke yourself with different types of touch–soft and slow, firm or hard.

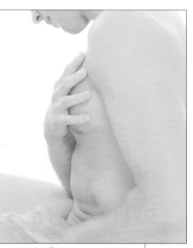

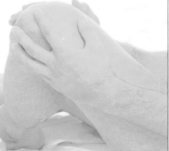

I'm a firm believer in massage exercises increasing sex drive. They also help us to tune into our sexual responses. But don't fall into the trap of feeling that from then on all sexual activity must lead to intercourse. At those times when one is longing for sex and the other doesn't feel like it, the less eager partner may be willing to massage his or her partner to climax.

STAGE ONE

Begin by concentrating completely on your own feelings. You want to awaken sensual feelings in yourself and learn what is arousing for you. Don't be hesitant about enhancing massage by trying it in a warm bath or bed.

Experiment with different kinds of stroking. All of these movements and sensations can be improved by using soap in the bath, and cream or body lotion in bed.

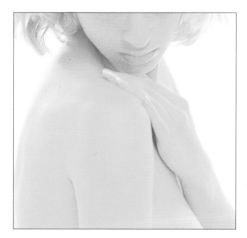

Massage yourself all over
Work from the top downward, if you like, until you feel fully in touch with your body's response to different sensations and you know how to arouse yourself. Do whatever feels good.

Concentrate on the sensations produced by your fingers against your skin

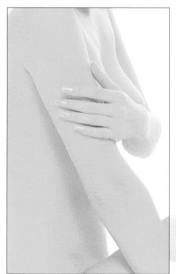

Experiment with different touches
Use the front and back of your hands, your fingertips and nails as you stroke upward and downward.

STAGE TWO

After a while, plan on involving your partner. Agree on a time when you can be undisturbed for some time, and can make adequate preparations such as having a bath together first, making sure the room is warm, having a relaxing drink, putting on some background music, getting the light just right — enough so that you can see each other — and then choose which one of you would like to start. You have to take turns.

Using a little cream or oil, massage and stroke each other all over, working your way down from head to toe, doing the back and then the front. Don't be afraid to show your pleasure at what feels

Concentrate on the pleasure your partner is giving you

good, and be very expressive and clear about your preferences. Try to keep your thoughts on how your body feels and verbalize them.

You should agree not to touch each other's genital areas the first few times you engage in mutual massage; take things very slowly and make sure that you are both comfortable and relaxed. Don't hurry the stages and don't give up. You may not see any benefits to your sex life immediately, but the massage will certainly feel deeply pleasurable, particularly if you concentrate on what is happening to your body, and what you are feeling now, at this minute.

Take it in turns

First you massage your partner, stroking him from head to toe all over. Let him enjoy each pleasurable sensation and express these feelings to you. Take things slowly! Then have your partner massage you. Be very clear about what feels good and gives you the most pleasure. Don't be concerned at all about the possible outcome; this is all about focusing your attention on what your body is feeling.

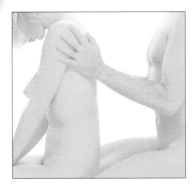

STAGE THREE

After another week or so, if both of you agree about the timing, you can move on to touching the more sexually sensitive parts of each other's body. Take each of the organs in turn. You should begin by showing each other how to give the most pleasure by the man stroking the breasts, the clitoris, the vagina, and the area near the anus, while the woman massages the penis, strokes the scrotum, and caresses his anal area. If your inclinations take you, you can go on from touching to kissing and licking, the only condition being that both of you should enjoy it. Another rule might be to talk, and to talk as much as you can; in fact, try to keep up a running commentary on how you are feeling, and describe how much you are enjoying the most pleasurable areas. During these sexual massages one of you may become more eager for orgasm than the other, but you should not have intercourse together before you both feel ready for it. It is the duty and the responsibility of the faster partner to wait for the slower one to catch up, and to make sure that the slower partner does catch up.

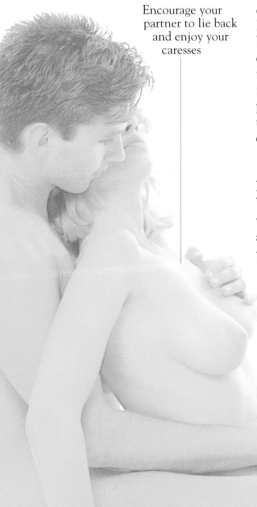

Encourage your partner to lie back and enjoy your caresses

Proceed at your own pace
When massage moves on to touching the woman's breasts, clitoris, and vaginal areas, and the man's more sexually sensitive parts, you will probably feel so highly stimulated that you will want to proceed to intercourse. This is fine provided you both feel comfortable doing so.

LACK OF ORGASM

No matter how sophisticated, attractive, or desirable a woman may be, she always faces the critical moment of truth: is she going to achieve orgasm or isn't she?

Very few women suffer from physiological orgasmic impairment; what they often suffer from is an impaired partner. He won't find out her preferences or needs, or is unaware how to stimulate her to bring her to orgasm. Of the women who do suffer from orgasmic impairment, many are tortured by a vague suspicion that every other woman in the world can always reach orgasm.

This, of course, is not true. Women often fail to achieve orgasm, and if you expect to reach orgasm every time you make love then your expectations are unrealistic. But every woman is capable of orgasm and can learn how to do it by masturbating (see page 74).

PAINFUL INTERCOURSE

It is quite common for a woman occasionally to experience some tightness in the entrance to the vagina or experience some pain or discomfort on intercourse. Painful intercourse, or dyspareunia, whatever the cause, has a common element in that it always involves some sort of pain in or around the vagina during intercourse. The pain may be deep and aching, sharp, a momentary twinge, or simply intense discomfort. The pain may be any combination of all these things, but it hurts, and though intercourse may proceed while the woman suffers, it cannot possibly be enjoyable for either party.

There are several possible reasons for painful intercourse, the most common being a clumsy or unsophisticated partner. Painful intercourse may result from infections and other disorders of the urinary tract, and, of course, much more rarely, there may be an anatomical defect that has been present since birth involving the size or shape of the vagina. Painful intercourse that is not the result of a medical disorder may be relieved by the following:

HOW A MAN CAN HELP

• Engage in adequate foreplay so that your partner is primed for intercourse and is stimulated so that she produces sufficient vaginal lubrication.

• Make sure you use a lubricant when attempting any form of penetration.

WHAT A WOMAN SHOULD DO

• Spread your thighs wide and bend your knees to facilitate entry.

• As your partner enters you, you should bear down slightly as if you are trying to push something out of your vagina. This will loosen up your vaginal muscles.

VAGINISMUS

Psychological factors can cause a muscle spasm of the vagina that causes the muscles around the entrance to close so tightly that intercourse becomes impossible. A woman has no control over this spasm; it is a reflex and therefore she cannot be blamed for it.

Women who have this problem may be otherwise sexually responsive but nearly all of them report a fear of intercourse or a past history of painful intercourse when they wished to avoid all sexual activity. Some women have had a very punitive or strict upbringing that leads them to believe that sexual intercourse, even with their husbands, is somehow evil or degrading. Some women feel guilty or just plain scared about voluntarily engaging in sex. A fear of becoming pregnant (which usually can be alleviated with appropriate contraception), can also lead to vaginismus in some women. If a woman has had an early frightening or dramatic experience with sexual intercourse she may also suffer from it. Women may have tried intercourse but failed because of a lack of lubrication. Others may have suffered from the trauma of being raped or sexually molested.

For some women, a first attempt at intercourse or a different position may be so unsuccessful, and produce so much anxiety, that they become progressively more nervous about the next attempt and experience vaginismus. All these causes can be treated.

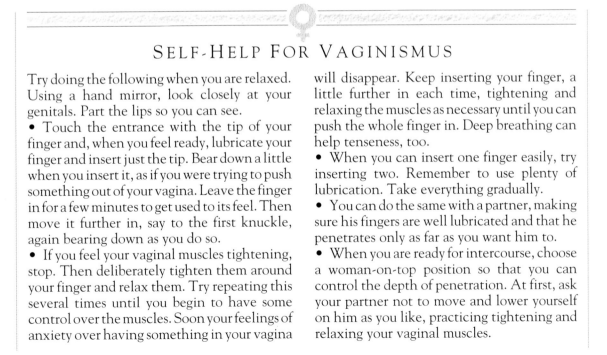

SELF-HELP FOR VAGINISMUS

Try doing the following when you are relaxed. Using a hand mirror, look closely at your genitals. Part the lips so you can see.

• Touch the entrance with the tip of your finger and, when you feel ready, lubricate your finger and insert just the tip. Bear down a little when you insert it, as if you were trying to push something out of your vagina. Leave the finger in for a few minutes to get used to its feel. Then move it further in, say to the first knuckle, again bearing down as you do so.

• If you feel your vaginal muscles tightening, stop. Then deliberately tighten them around your finger and relax them. Try repeating this several times until you begin to have some control over the muscles. Soon your feelings of anxiety over having something in your vagina will disappear. Keep inserting your finger, a little further in each time, tightening and relaxing the muscles as necessary until you can push the whole finger in. Deep breathing can help tenseness, too.

• When you can insert one finger easily, try inserting two. Remember to use plenty of lubrication. Take everything gradually.

• You can do the same with a partner, making sure his fingers are well lubricated and that he penetrates only as far as you want him to.

• When you are ready for intercourse, choose a woman-on-top position so that you can control the depth of penetration. At first, ask your partner not to move and lower yourself on him as you like, practicing tightening and relaxing your vaginal muscles.

MEN'S PROBLEMS

Probably the most frequent problem men have with ejaculations is having them before they are wanted. The term premature ejaculation is often attached to this situation, which is better expressed as a problem in achieving proper timing of ejaculation or achieving a reasonable amount of control over it.

However, as men get older they sometimes get upset that it takes too long to ejaculate. Indeed, some older men may not be able to ejaculate at all from time to time. Some men and their partners get upset about it, others just take it in stride as one more slowing down process among many.

Some older men even find enjoyment in a less intense, more relaxed pattern of sexuality, and don't consider speedy ejaculation to be essential for enjoying themselves. Men should remember that the most enjoyable sexual encounters are not goal-oriented; ejaculation can be a satisfying and natural climax to lovemaking, but if it becomes the only goal, or even the major goal of a man, much of the joy of sexual contact may be lost for him as well as for his partner.

Over the age of 40, nearly all men are anxious about their abilities to maintain erections. Even if a man has never experienced difficulties with erection, he feels that impotence due to poor erection is a hazard of aging. Probably, the fallacy that impotence is to be expected as a man ages is more firmly entrenched in our culture than almost any other sexual myth.

PREMATURE EJACULATION

Problems of premature ejaculation disturb mostly younger men. For them, fears of performance are not due to problems of erection but with the inability to control their ejaculations sufficiently to satisfy their female partners.

Men with a tendency to premature ejaculation are more numerous than is generally assumed, but this major handicap sometimes disappears with age. As a man gets used to making love with the same woman, he exercises better self-control or more suitable sexual techniques. If the problem persists, then its origins are deeper, but it is usually easily cured with professional help.

A better name for premature ejaculation might be "immature ejaculation." No one is sure what causes such ejaculatory enthusiasm, and it is certainly possible that some men have more rapid reflexes than others. Learning experiences in adolescence may condition some men to have rapid ejaculations: men who suffer from this condition are unwittingly perpetuating their original patterns of adolescent masturbation. When they were 14 years old, the idea was to apply friction to the penis as rapidly and as intensely as possible and then ejaculate.

Premature ejaculation is the result of a temporary or permanent fault in the process of sexual arousal; the penis has a normal erection and reaches its maximum size at the moment of ejaculation. Ejaculation is premature when it occurs as soon as the glans touches the vulva, penetrates the vagina, or as often happens, as a result of the caresses made during foreplay, even before any attempt at penetration. Immediately after ejaculation, the penis becomes limp again and returns to its former size.

Premature ejaculation can be a serious problem in normal intercourse, much to both partners' dismay and confusion. It generally occurs in nervous, highly emotional men; it can occur often in men who are victims of a narrow education or of socio-religious taboos. Premature ejaculation can occur also after a prolonged period of abstinence, or in the presence of a new partner, or some extraordinary stimulation. However, there are ways to alleviate the problem.

HOW TO HOLD BACK EJACULATION   Techniques for solving the problem of premature ejaculation involve the full cooperation of the woman, as well as the man. A man should always discuss any "exercises" with his partner so she's relaxed, informed, and enthusiastic about sharing them. Both of them should be agreed about what they will do, like experimenting with positions in order to find those in which the man can best control ejaculation.

WHAT A MAN SHOULD DO

• Block your mind from thinking about sex and use distraction techniques.
• Limit foreplay to an absolute minimum and avoid touching your partner's sex organs.
• Place the penis in your partner's vagina very carefully, avoiding too much stimulation.
• Keep thrusting movements to a minimum, because keeping the penis motionless is the best way to control the ejaculatory reflex.
• Occasionally withdraw your penis from your partner's vagina.
• Inhale very deeply and tighten your abdominal muscles at the point of ejaculation.
• Exhale your breath once the urge to ejaculate passes.

HOW A WOMAN CAN HELP

• Remain deliberately passive; do not contract your vaginal muscles around your partner's penis or move your pelvis at all.
• Keep visual and olfactory stimulation to a minimum by wearing unsexy nightclothes and not using perfume.
• Encourage your partner to make love several times in succession; this can produce some control even if he ejaculates prematurely but is better from then on.
• Suggest making love at times when your partner is tired and his arousal is low; this may delay ejaculation correspondingly. Other good times to try are when he wakes up, since he may have an asexual erection.

ABSENCE OF EJACULATION

THE MAN'S EXPERIENCE   This man normally enjoys a healthy and satisfying sex life. He works very hard and enjoys relaxing with his present long-term partner. However, on returning from a tiring business trip he found that he felt highly excited but could not reach orgasm while making love. This caused him some anxiety as it had only happened to him once before when he was very drunk. However, after resting, he and his partner started to make love again; this time he had no problems reaching a climax and ejaculating in the normal way.

ORGASM

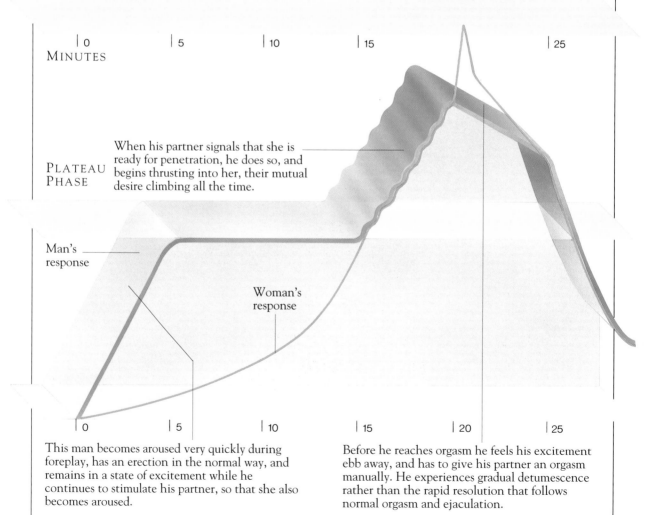

0   30
Normal pattern
Absence of ejaculation

MINUTES | 0 | 5 | 10 | 15 | 25

PLATEAU
PHASE

When his partner signals that she is ready for penetration, he does so, and begins thrusting into her, their mutual desire climbing all the time.

Man's response

Woman's response

0   5   10   15   20   25

This man becomes aroused very quickly during foreplay, has an erection in the normal way, and remains in a state of excitement while he continues to stimulate his partner, so that she also becomes aroused.

Before he reaches orgasm he feels his excitement ebb away, and has to give his partner an orgasm manually. He experiences gradual detumescence rather than the rapid resolution that follows normal orgasm and ejaculation.

TOO RAPID EJACULATION

THE MAN'S EXPERIENCE   This man has a regular sex life with his partner, whom he has known for some years. He always initiates sex because he believes that a man has a strong physical need to have sex whereas women don't, and he doesn't seem to mind that his partner is never very keen. He likes to have sex in what he calls "the old-fashioned way" – in a fast, passionate burst of activity so that his partner doesn't know what's hit her. He has always found it much more exciting that way, and thinks that women like to be dominated in bed or they don't respect you.

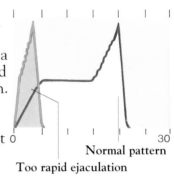

Normal pattern

Too rapid ejaculation

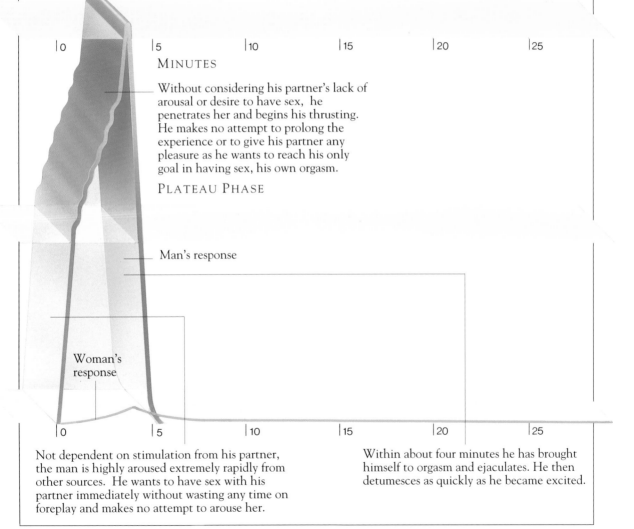

ORGASM

|0 |5 |10 |15 |20 |25

MINUTES

Without considering his partner's lack of arousal or desire to have sex, he penetrates her and begins his thrusting. He makes no attempt to prolong the experience or to give his partner any pleasure as he wants to reach his only goal in having sex, his own orgasm.

PLATEAU PHASE

Man's response

Woman's response

|0 |5 |10 |15 |20 |25

Not dependent on stimulation from his partner, the man is highly aroused extremely rapidly from other sources. He wants to have sex with his partner immediately without wasting any time on foreplay and makes no attempt to arouse her.

Within about four minutes he has brought himself to orgasm and ejaculates. He then detumesces as quickly as he became excited.

PREMATURE EJACULATION

THE MAN'S EXPERIENCE   This man cannot enjoy
prolonged sexual intercourse with his partner because he
does not have sufficient control over his reflexes. He
ejaculates too soon and abruptly interrupts lovemaking.
Sometimes, if he and his partner have an extended period
of foreplay, he loses control and ejaculates before he has
even penetrated her. At other times the first few thrusts
are enough to cause him to ejaculate. Despite the fact that
he reaches orgasm, it is not very pleasurable.

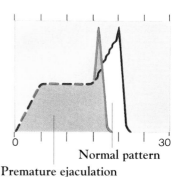

Normal pattern

Premature ejaculation

ORGASM

| 0 | 5

MINUTES

At other times, he is able to penetrate his partner but despite all his
efforts to prolong her arousal, after
the first few thrusts, he ejaculates,
unable to control the stimulation
intercourse produces.

PLATEAU PHASE

Man's
response

Woman's
response

| 0 | 5 | 10 | 15 | 20 | 25

The man becomes excited very quickly and stays at the
plateau phase for only a few minutes during foreplay,
wanting to fully stimulate his partner while trying to keep
his own arousal in check. Sometimes, however, the
excitement of foreplay is enough to cause him to ejaculate.

THE WOMAN'S EXPERIENCE The woman tries to be understanding about her partner's problem but cannot help feeling despondent and frustrated at the lack of pleasure both of them derive from their lovemaking. She appreciates that her partner tries to stimulate her before penetration, but hates not being able to explore and touch his body, since even a little stimulation proves to be too much. When they do get as far as intercourse, he climaxes within a few seconds and the experience feels empty for both of them.

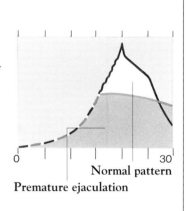

Normal pattern

Premature ejaculation

ORGASM

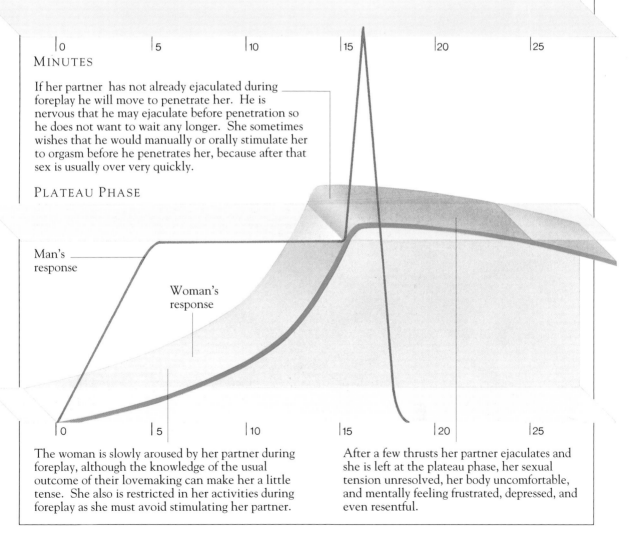

MINUTES

If her partner has not already ejaculated during foreplay he will move to penetrate her. He is nervous that he may ejaculate before penetration so he does not want to wait any longer. She sometimes wishes that he would manually or orally stimulate her to orgasm before he penetrates her, because after that sex is usually over very quickly.

PLATEAU PHASE

Man's response

Woman's response

The woman is slowly aroused by her partner during foreplay, although the knowledge of the usual outcome of their lovemaking can make her a little tense. She also is restricted in her activities during foreplay as she must avoid stimulating her partner.

After a few thrusts her partner ejaculates and she is left at the plateau phase, her sexual tension unresolved, her body uncomfortable, and mentally feeling frustrated, depressed, and even resentful.

HOW TO HOLD BACK EJACULATION (CONT'D)   Along with the squeeze technique (below), the man should practice controlling his ejaculatory reflex by regularly holding back; all men can achieve this. With his partner's active help a man can learn to use the following three-step method:

1 Have intercourse without stimulation or ejaculation.

2 Have intercourse with stimulation but without ejaculation.

3 Have controlled and prolonged intercourse without stimulation and ejaculation.

Controlling the ejaculatory reflex naturally needs considerable practice – more for some than others – but once it is achieved it will result in great personal satisfaction. Again, as with other sexual therapy, it is imperative to have a partner's compliance in any of the exercises that you will undertake.

THE SQUEEZE TECHNIQUE

This is a procedure developed by Masters and Johnson designed to retrain the brain to control ejaculatory reflex. It can be done by either the man alone, or with his partner. If a man is able to delay ejaculation regularly, he becomes increasingly confident that he can successfully maintain a state of sexual arousal without having to have an immediate orgasm.

Sex therapists normally supervise couples in this therapy, but it's easy enough to attempt without specialist treatment.

Initially the woman stimulates her partner's penis until he has an erection. He will want to ejaculate, but to stop this from happening, she is told to press the tip of his penis for a few seconds by placing her thumb on his frenulum, and her first and second fingers on the ridge of the glans on its upper side. When he advises her that his urge to ejaculate has gone, she should start caressing him again.

Each time that he feels he is on the point of ejaculating, the man signals and the woman starts the squeeze technique again. This procedure can be kept up for 15 to 20 minutes until the man decides he must have an orgasm. At the beginning of the training process, inter-

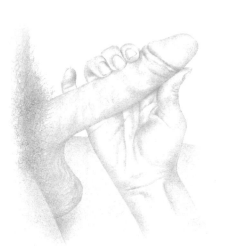

Grasping the Penis
The woman squeezes the penis, gripping with her thumb and forefinger just below the glans, and presses gently for ten seconds, or firmly for five seconds. One or two hands can be used.

course should be limited to only a few minutes; then, as a man's self-control improves, the duration can be increased gradually. Also, it is best if the man's bladder is completely empty before attempting any of the exercises.

—— DIFFICULTIES WITH ERECTIONS ——

Spontaneous or asexual erections, which all men and even young boys experience, occur without the slightest erotic stimulation, and are simply a sign that the erection system is working well. They can be produced, for instance, by the vibrations during a car or train journey, by the rhythm of a regular movement such as bicycle riding or horseback riding, by compression of the penis when a man is sitting or lying, by the congestion of his abdomen during the digestive process, or on his waking up in the morning stretched out in a warm bed. These early morning erections, like all other spontaneous erections, appear to follow the curve of sexual vitality, and their frequency decreases with age.

The frequency of erections is not the only thing that changes with age. As a man gets older his erection is no longer as upright. The penis gradually stops becoming as hard as it did when he was young, and nearly all men have difficulty maintaining an erection once they are in their fifties. Some may notice an earlier decline, say from 45 years.

PUTTING PROBLEMS INTO PERSPECTIVE It's important that such impotence always be viewed merely as a temporary setback in the development of an active sex life. Any man, even the strongest, most competent, and most virile, however old he is, will, at some point in his life, experience a breakdown of his system. A man would not create a fuss if it were only a question of losing his sexual desire or feeling completely indifferent toward his partner; the drama lies in the man thinking that this moment of failure is a permanent disability — although in general, it is only a brief occasional or temporary problem nearly always psychological in origin. The main emotions that induce impotence are fear, guilt, and anxiety.

All men grow up believing that the essence of a man's sexual potency is expressed by his ability to have an erection whenever he feels aroused, introduce a rigid penis into a woman's vagina, keep it there, and ejaculate at orgasm. In short, his capacity to have sex at any time, in any place, just when he chooses.

All too often a man at any age, but mainly as he's getting older, considerably exaggerates the importance of sex over all other aspects of a relationship. One day when he discovers that he cannot get an erection, he experiences a moment of fear, something like the disintegration of a power he thought had no limits.

The whole point is that if a man should, for any reason, find he is momentarily impotent he still can give his partner complete satisfaction in bed. Intercourse is only one of a hundred different ways in which a woman can reach an orgasm. Recognizing this can take the pressure off of both partners.

An impotent man who has acquired enough confidence to become expert at various caresses can be a perfect lover. He will be able to produce orgasm of a rare quality and of a different intensity than those provoked by the penis, which is a much less precise organ than the tongue or a finger.

A sexually fulfilled woman will not be at all disappointed in a partner with a declining erection if he skillfully makes up for this by using a variety of methods to satisfy her desires.

ACHIEVING AN ERECTION The majority of men, however, would still like to enjoy an erection, and there are several ways that they and their partners can go about making it more likely that they do so. When impotence is of long standing, specialist attention (see opposite) may be needed.

WHAT A MAN SHOULD DO

• Psychologically prepare yourself by telling yourself that from now on you're not going to be impotent.
• Discuss any emotional problems with your partner and talk through them.
• Be in good sexual condition, which means be in good physical condition and at a normal weight.
• Ascertain that the impotence is not a result of a disease such as diabetes, multiple sclerosis, or atherosclerosis.
• Stop taking all drugs including alcohol, nicotine, sleeping pills, tranquilizers, painkillers, etc. — everything that is not prescribed. If you are taking prescription drugs, ask your doctor whether they are capable of causing impotence and if so, whether alternatives are available.
• Attempt sexual intercourse even when the penis is not erect, because sexual intercourse is the most powerful sexual stimulant.
• Try various mechanical devices, like a vibrator with a suction-cuplike attachment which, once lubricated, is applied gently to the head of the penis.
• In persistent cases, ask about penile implants or injections (see opposite page).

HOW A WOMAN CAN HELP

• Passionate, intelligent, and enlightened foreplay of the penis, including gentle stroking with the fingertips from the base to the tip, followed by massage of the frenulum and the glans, and alternate squeezing and massaging of the shaft, should trigger erectile response in your partner.
• Offer positive sexual reinforcement if your partner manages to penetrate you but loses his erection before either you or he has an orgasm.
• Gently twist the part of the glans that lies between the crown and the tip using your thumb and forefinger.
• Pinch the frenulum gently between your fingers; this can be a little painful but usually produces a sudden reaction that makes the penis stiffen.
• Form a ring with your thumb and forefinger and gently squeeze the top of the penis just beneath the frenulum. This prevents venous drainage from the penis and it becomes stiffer very quickly.

LONG-LASTING IMPOTENCE

Up until a few years ago, most doctors believed that lasting impotence in the majority of men who suffered from it was due to psychological problems. However, it is now known that impotence is frequently the result of an illness, taking certain drugs, or damage caused by an accident that interferes with the nerve supply to the pelvis. For older men, the most likely cause is atherosclerosis, the clogging of the arteries caused by smoking and a diet rich in fat.

These discoveries about the causes of impotence led to advances in treatment. The first was when a French doctor discovered that injections of drugs into the penis could artificially induce erections, and recently, an advanced surgical method for the treatment of impotence with a penile implant has become more widespread.

An alternative treatment to surgery for men who are healthy enough to have a good blood supply to the penis is an injection of papaverine into a groin artery. This results in erection, though the response is unpredictable in some men and can last a long time. If an erection lasts more than four hours, medical attention will be needed. Often a low-dose injection is all that is necessary to increase responsiveness, and injections may not be required all the time. Talk to your doctor if you feel you're suffering from long-term impotence.

PENILE IMPLANT

There are various types of penile implants; the type shown here gives complete control over erection and remains a permanent fixture.

It consists of two inflatable rods that are surgically installed in the penis. The rods are inserted into the corpora cavernosa, which normally fill with blood when a man has an erection. These are inflated hydraulically by a little pump, placed in the scrotum, which draws fluid from a reservoir inserted in the abdomen. This makes the penis rigid.

After intercourse, a man can deflate his penis by pressing a small button attached to the pump. The rods are of a fixed length, which means that the penis remains extended even when the rods are deflated, but the penis will be soft enough to fold away. A man is not aware of the pump in his scrotum except when he feels for it there.

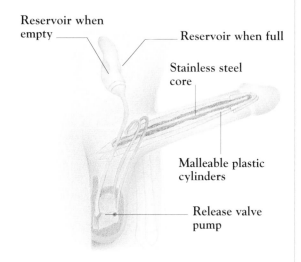

Reservoir when empty

Reservoir when full

Stainless steel core

Malleable plastic cylinders

Release valve pump

A permanent implant
This enables the penis to become rigid via a pump inserted in the abdomen.

EMOTIONAL FACTORS

It should be clear to anyone reading the preceding pages that most sexual problems are the result of emotional disparities between partners. If a man has a fear of disappointing a woman, being abandoned by her, or has any ambivalence toward her, this can prevent him from letting go during sex and push him toward becoming nonejaculatory in bed.

If a woman feels disappointment because her partner has ignored her feelings, bored because he doesn't produce an orgasm for her, or angry that he doesn't seem to care if she is sexually satisfied, she can become unresponsive in bed. And both men and women can become preoccupied by work problems, or social and family life, which can prevent them from devoting sufficient attention to lovemaking. Fatigue, failure to eat and exercise, sleep disruption, or poor performance at work also can impair sexual reflexes.

I believe that the majority of cases where problems suddenly arise over a temporary situation can be solved without a therapist, as long as a partner is loving and responsive. Usually just talking over the problem, preferably out of bed so there is no direct link between sexual performance and what is under discussion, can cure most of these setbacks. It also helps to return to courtship behavior, which is intimate without being too pressured.

Bear in mind, too, that a nonsexist attitude is essential for a good sexual relationship so that each partner has equal standing within the relationship and all activities are open to both. If either partner sees the other as having a preassigned sex role, then an artificial and destructive limit can be placed on sexual intimacy.

— GRIEF DEPRESSES SEXUAL FEELING —

Not surprisingly, sex is adversely affected by bereavement. Grief almost certainly has a distinct and traceable impact — not only on sexual relationships but on simple intimacy. Some bereaved people may impose on themselves a compensatory celibacy, a sort of paying the penance for imaginary or real responsibility for the loss. Feelings of love for a partner may be lost, as will libido and an awareness of the sexual attractiveness of the other.

Grieving is a de-energizing process, and a bereaved partner feels weak, withdrawn, and listless; he or she may also feel that personal sexual attractiveness has been lost. There is a period during which self-care, attention to hygiene, dressing, posture, and presentation are ignored or neglected. A bereaved person may present this "grieving mask" to avoid intimacy and to hide from insensitive sexual overtures.

REPRODUCTION, CONTRA-CEPTION, AND SEXUALLY TRANSMITTED DISEASE

WHAT YOU NEED TO KNOW

The biological reason for human sex is reproduction, to ensure the continued existence and development of the species. Human beings are unique in the extent to which they enjoy not just intercourse but a wide range of other sexual activities, and the way in which they can separate the pleasurable act of sex from the function of reproduction.

Reproduction is a fascinatingly complex process, involving the fertilization of a woman's egg by a man's sperm and the subsequent development of the microscopically small fertilized egg into a human baby. But to separate sex from reproduction, some form of contraception is necessary so that intercourse does not result in pregnancy.

Contraception takes many forms. They vary in their effectiveness, their ease of use, and their possible side effects, but every couple should be able to find a contraceptive method that suits their particular needs. One of the simplest methods of effective contraception — the condom or sheath — has been in use for centuries, but it fell out of favor in the 1960s and 1970s when less intrusive contraceptives, in the form of the Pill and the IUD, became available. Recently, however, the condom has been making a comeback, partly because of its lack of potentially harmful side effects and partly because of its ability to protect both partners from many forms of sexually transmitted disease, especially AIDS.

AIDS, Acquired Immune Deficiency Syndrome, is caused by the Human Immunodeficiency Virus (HIV) and it was first recognized as a specific condition in 1981. Its origins are still unknown, and because there is, as yet, no cure for it, the only wise course of action for an individual is to practice "safe sex" and avoid indulging in activities that carry a risk of exposure to HIV.

In comparison with the ultimately fatal AIDS, the other sexually transmitted diseases are relatively harmless. But they are all unpleasant, and many can lead to serious complications, including death, if treatment is delayed or neglected. Any genital pain, discomfort, discharge, blisters, lumps, or sores should receive prompt medical attention from a doctor.

Consultations and treatment are totally confidential, but it is essential that anyone who contracts a sexually transmitted disease should inform their partner or partners so that they too can seek treatment, and also avoid passing the disease on to others.

This is especially important in the case of female partners, because some diseases can be symptomless in women. If a woman is not told that her partner may have infected her, the disease might cause her serious problems before it becomes apparent that she has it, and before treatment can begin.

REPRODUCTION

If couples have intercourse without contraception, eight out of ten women will be pregnant within a year: 25 percent of them will conceive within one month, 60 percent within six months and 75 percent within nine months. Within eighteen months, 90 percent of women having unprotected intercourse will become pregnant. The number of conceptions becomes progressively smaller with time until finally, less than ten percent of couples are left childless.

Female fertility is fairly low immediately after puberty and reaches a peak about the age of 24; it begins to decline after the age of 30. The effects of the woman's age on fertility are complex; advancing age brings with it less frequent ovulation, irregularities in the progestergenic phase of her cycle, an increasingly unfavorable uterine environment, and diminished chances of survival of her ova. The effects of age on men are less critical, and while fertility has been recorded at 94 years of age, it does begin to decline after age 24.

It is not possible to know whether or not an individual is fertile without specialist examination; a woman can tell if she is ovulating by keeping a daily temperature chart and noting its rise, but this doesn't tell her anything about the transport of the ovum or about its implanting successfully. Even if the ejaculate looks normal, there is no way of knowing that it contains the right number or kind of sperm.

— WHAT REPRODUCTION INVOLVES —

During sexual intercourse, up to five hundred million sperm are ejaculated into the vagina. Many of them leak out again and only about two thousand survive the journey through the cervix and into the uterus to reach the Fallopian tubes. When sperm hit the comparatively enormous ovum (egg), they attach themselves over its entire surface and, driven by their tails, attempt to penetrate the ovum. However, only one sperm pierces the outer coat of the ovum. Instantly, the egg loses its attraction, hardens its outer shell, and all the superfluous sperm let go. This whole process of ejaculation to fertilization usually takes less than 60 minutes.

Once the ovum is fertilized, it begins to divide and multiply while it continues its journey through the Fallopian tube. Eventually it will implant itself in the uterine wall and proceed to develop into a fetus.

Before insemination and fertilization can take place, however, sperm must gain access to an ovum. This involves a number of complicated transport problems in both male and female genital tracts — from the seminiferous tubules in the testes to the ampullae of the Fallopian tubes, a journey described on the following pages.

THE MAN'S CONTRIBUTION

The transport, maturation, and maintenance of sperm are the most important functions of the male reproductive tract.

Newly formed sperm pass from the seminiferous tubules of each testis to a system of coiled tubes, the epididymis, that is connected to it. There they will mature. As they leave the testes, sperm are nonmobile and incapable of fertilizing an ovum. They need modification before they can fertilize an ovum, and once this modification is completed, sperm enter a long tube called the vas deferens which, with its smooth muscular coat, propels them into the ejaculatory tract to collect in secondary storage sites called ampullae.

A SPERM'S STRUCTURE

Each sperm is tadpole-shaped and about 60 microns (a micron is a thousandth of a millimeter) long or .00024 inch, and its head is flattened, pear-shaped, and compressed at the front into a flat edge.

The sperm head is composed almost entirely of a nucleus densely packed with DNA; each sperm contains its own selection of genetic material. The head is protected by a caplike structure, or acrosome, which contains enzymes that help the sperm penetrate the wall of the ovum during fertilization. The sperm retains its "cap" until it reaches the ovum and then sheds it, possibly because of substances the ovum has produced.

The sperm represents the genetic contribution to a baby from the father, and the nucleus contains 23 chromosomes. When a sperm unites with an ovum, the resulting cell has the full complement of 46 chromosomes: 23 from the father and 23 from the mother.

The tail of a sperm is joined to the head by a short neck, and whiplike movements of the tail allow the sperm to travel to reach the ovum moving through the Fallopian tube. A sperm takes about 64 days to be fully formed, and must be maintained at a temperature several degrees lower than that of the abdominal cavity. Even a slight elevation in the temperature of the testes can result in a transient impairment of sperm production.

INSEMINATION

Insemination, or the method by which semen is naturally deposited in the vagina, involves three reflexes — erection, emission, and ejaculation. All the reflexes occur at the level of the spinal cord and are moderated by impulses from the brain.

The penis must be erect for penetration of the vagina, and the essential factor in penile erection is dilation (expansion) of the arteries carrying the blood supply to the penis. When these arteries are fully dilated, they close off the veins that carry the blood away from the penis. Thus the penis becomes swollen with more and more blood, which cannot escape, and therefore becomes erect.

When a man becomes sexually aroused, sperm from the ampullae and fluid from the nearby seminal vesicles are pumped down to the urethra, a process known as emission. The nerve impulses that initiate this process are carried from touch receptors in the glans penis.

Ejaculation is the propulsion of semen and seminal fluid out of the urethra, and is triggered by the same stimuli that induce emission. Impulses from the touch receptors in the glans penis cause rhythmic contractions of the urethra and the prostate, a gland at the beginning of the urethra.

The prostate secretes a nutrient fluid that becomes part of the seminal plasma, and muscular contractions pump the ejaculate outward; the internal bladder sphincter, a circular muscle around the exit of the bladder, closes to prevent ejaculate from entering the bladder and to stop urine from leaving it. The volume of the ejaculate ranges from 1 to 5 ml (from one-quarter to just over a teaspoon), of which only ten percent is sperm; the other 90 percent is composed of the seminal plasma.

Most young men can ejaculate several times a day and middle-aged men can manage two or three times. It is only in old age that things appear to "dry up" and semen volume falls.

THE SPERM'S JOURNEY

During intercourse, sperm are ejaculated into a woman's vagina. The journey of 6 to 7 inches (about 15 to 18 cms), the approximate distance from vagina to Fallopian tube, generally takes several hours.

During the sperm's ascent of the woman's genital tract there is an enormous reduction in sperm number. As many as five hundred million sperm are ejaculated with the initial reduction occurring at the cervix; it is filled with mucus that can be impassable, and lined with recesses into which many sperm disappear.

White blood corpuscles present in the woman's body can also kill sperm, especially if she has any infection. Further elimination occurs at the junction with the uterine tubes so that only a couple of thousand sperm enter the tubes, and only about one or two hundred sperm penetrate further.

While the sperm have made this journey, they themselves have been changed by substances in the cervix and Fallopian tubes, so that those that reach the ovum should have become capacitated, capable of fertilization.

FERTILIZATION OR NOT

An ovum does not attract sperm; sperm simply swim past, and if they hit it, they begin to push their heads into the egg's walls, driven by their beating tails. The cap of the sperm releases enzymes that strip the egg of its nutrient cells. When the egg's surface is completely exposed, one of the remaining sperm penetrates the ovum's inner cell plasma. As soon as this happens, the chemical composition of the egg's wall changes, and it shuts out all other sperm, even ones that have partially penetrated it. The leftover sperm continue to agitate around the egg, or if there was no egg at all, they swim back and forth in the tube.

Sperm may remain fertile and mobile in the female tract for one to two days, but the ripe ovum can probably survive for only 12 to 24 hours. Therefore, fertilization is unlikely unless intercourse occurs one or two days before or immediately after ovulation.

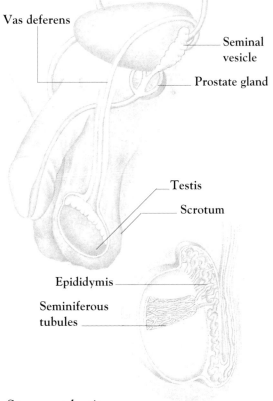

Sperm production
In a phenomenal feat of creation, many millions of sperm are formed daily. They are created in the seminiferous tubules, millions of tiny, tubular structures within the testes.

FERTILIZATION

Sperm, following intercourse and ejaculation, swim up through the cervix toward the Fallopian tubes. Once in the tube, they surround the egg and attempt to penetrate it until one is successful. The union of an ovum and a sperm creates a zygote, and is known as the process of fertilization.

Following fertilization, the zygote begins cell division, becoming a blastocyst, and continues down the Fallopian tube into the uterus where it implants itself in the uterine wall.

Sperm meet the egg

Mature ovum

Ovary

Fallopian tube

The ovarian cycle

Each month of a woman's life while she is fertile, the pituitary gland in the brain secretes follicle stimulating hormone (FSH), which stimulates (usually) one of the ovaries to grow an egg follicle. A woman's ova, or eggs, are stored in the follicles, and these ripen inside. When there are sufficient levels of FSH hormone, and another hormone, luteinizing hormone, in circulation, the follicle bursts and releases the egg into the Fallopian tube—the process known as ovulation. The egg is then carried down the tube toward the uterus, where as a fertilized egg it implants itself in the uterine wall (a pregnancy), or as an unfertilized egg, it is expelled, along with the uterine lining, during menstruation. The follicle that housed the egg matures into a corpus luteum, which secretes large amounts of progesterone in the second half of the month. This then ages and dies.

The blastocyst
The blastocyst is the ball of cells created by the cell division within the fertilized ovum. It travels through the Fallopian tube, continuing to divide until it reaches the uterus, approximately seven days after fertilization.

Uterus

Location of the female reproductive tract

Boy or Girl?

A baby's sex is determined by the sex chromosomes found in the man's sperm. A woman's ovum is female and contains only X chromosomes. Sperm can be male or female. A boy is produced when a sperm containing a Y chromosome penetrates the ovum; a girl is produced when a sperm containing an X chromosome combines with the ovum.

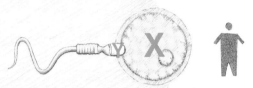

Y sperm plus X ovum equals XY chromosome, or a male

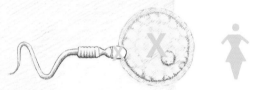

X sperm plus X ovum equals XX chromosome, or a female

Twins

At the time of ovulation, a change in information sent to the ovary by the brain and pituitary gland can result in more than one ovum being released enabling fraternal (nonidentical) twins or triplets to be conceived, each with its own placenta. This tendency often runs in families. However, if a single fertilized egg divides into two equal parts, identical twins result.

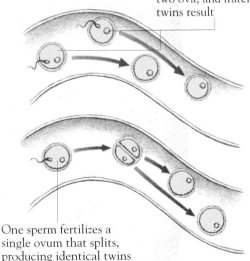

Two sperm fertilize two ova, and fraternal twins result

One sperm fertilizes a single ovum that splits, producing identical twins

THE WOMAN'S CONTRIBUTION

The organs that enable a woman to produce mature ova, transport them to be fertilized, and then nourish the fertilized eggs, are all found within the pelvic cavity.

THE OVARIES

The two ovaries, the organs that produce the eggs, are flattened bean-shaped glands about 1½ inches long, ¾-inch wide, and ½-inch thick. Their surface is pearly white, and their contours are wrinkled.

The position of the ovaries in the pelvis is variable, but in women who have borne no children they lie on the side of the pelvic walls with their long axes vertical. Their inner sides lie toward the pelvic cavity but are overhung by the uterine tubes. The ovaries are supported on three sides by ligaments.

An ovary is made up of two layers — the outer cortex from which the ova emerge, and the center, called the medulla.

The ovaries play a central role in female reproduction and perform two intimately related functions: the production of ova and the production of sex hormones. These two functions are regulated by two centers in the brain — the hypothalamus and the adenohypophysis. In turn, the principal site of action for the ovarian hormones is the uterus, and ovulation may be followed by implantation of the fertilized ovum in the uterine cavity.

THE OVARIAN CYCLE

Both ovulation and the production of hormones by the ovary follow a strictly repetitive sequence — the ovarian cycle. This cycle is based on the growth changes around the female germ cells that produce ova. A woman's entire stock of germ cells is present in her ovaries when she is born. Each ovary contains about three to four million germ cells, although there is wide individual variation.

Less than one percent of these cells are destined to mature and be ovulated during the 35 years or so of her reproductive life. The rest simply shrivel away, a process which begins before birth and continues until menopause when the stock of germ cells is virtually exhausted.

Each month, some of these germ cells are surrounded by single layers of cells, forming structures called primordial follicles. The mechanism by which a single follicle matures each month is unknown, but it becomes less efficient with advancing years.

At the beginning of any month, several follicles may begin to develop, under the influence of follicle stimulating hormone (FSH) secreted by the pituitary gland; but only one (or occasionally two) continues to develop and the others regress.

The developing follicle matures during the first two weeks of a menstrual cycle. The mature follicle is known as the Graafian follicle and has a diameter of 10 to 30 mm — a thousand times bigger than the original primordial follicle from which it developed.

When the follicle reaches maturity, luteinizing hormone secreted by the pituitary gland causes it to rupture as it emerges on to the surface of the ovary. As it does so, it discharges the germ cell or ovum. Tiny, fringelike projections called fimbriae, at the end of each Fallopian tube, are close to the surface of the ovary and waft the ejected ovum into one of the tubes. Muscular contraction of the tube's wall then carries the ovum along to the ampulla, where it awaits fertilization by a sperm.

Following ovulation, the follicle collapses and becomes a corpus luteum, an intense yellow-colored body that actively synthesizes sex hormones for eight to ten days. Then, if fertilization has not occurred, it undergoes a process of degeneration and, over the next few months, degenerates into a structureless white mass called a corpus albicans.

THE OVUM

Ovulation occurs at the midpoint of each ovarian cycle and each ovum represents the genetic contribution of the mother to her baby. A child, however, is not simply the sum of a half share of maternal and paternal chromosomes. The chromosomes that it inherits at fertilization are similar to, but not identical with, parental chromosomes.

During the production of an ovum, the actual genetic structure of the chromosome from the mother's cells is rearranged so that the chromosomes in the ovum are genetically dissimilar to the corresponding chromosomes of the mother's tissues.

Fertilization involves the fusion of an ovum with a sperm. Therefore, in order to maintain the constancy of the number of human chromosome cells, the number of chromosomes in the ovum is reduced by half prior to fertilization, and becomes 23 rather than 46. This is achieved by two successive cell divisions known collectively as meiosis.

THE UTERUS

The uterus is a pear-shaped organ whose narrow end projects into the vagina. The upper two-thirds constitutes the body, and that portion of the body that lies above the junction with the uterine tubes is known as the fundus. The upper lateral angles where the tubes enter are known as the cornua. The lower one-third of the uterus is the cervix.

The nonpregnant uterus is flattened in a front to back direction, weighs about 1¾ to 3½ oz. (50 to 100 grams) and is about 3 inches long, 2 inches wide, and 1 inch thick (8 x 5 x 3 cms). It contains a muscular lining, the myometrium.

The uterus is slightly angled toward the right-hand side and, when viewed from the side, it is slightly bent forward on itself, although in about ten percent of women it is angled backward. The cervix meets the vagina at an angle of about 90 degrees.

The position of the uterus is affected by whether or not the bladder and rectum are adequately supported. Normally, when a woman stands erect, the cervix is at the level of the front pelvic bones. If, however, the pelvic muscles become weakened, the uterus may prolapse (drop down) well below this level.

The myometrium consists of bundles of smooth muscle fibers separated by connective tissue. These bundles are arranged in poorly defined layers but the bulk of muscle forms an interrelating network of fibers.

The mucus lining of the uterus, the endometrium, lies directly on top of the myometrium so that the tips of the endometrial glands may burrow into the underlying muscle. During the reproductive years, the endometrium undergoes cyclical changes.

THE FALLOPIAN TUBES

Each Fallopian or uterine tube is approximately 4 inches (10 cms) long. At its inner end, the tube is linked to the uterine cavity; its outer end opens into the pelvic cavity. Each tube has four parts. The first, the interstitial part, runs obliquely through the uterine muscle and leads to a narrow muscular region known as the isthmus. This is followed by a heavily folded segment called the ampulla. The outer end of each tube widens to form the infundibulum which is fringed by a number of long, tentacle-like structures called the fimbriae.

Some of the cells lining the Fallopian tubes are covered with hairlike projections that move sequentially, very much like a field of corn in the wind. These rippling movements are designed to carry ova from the ovaries into the tubes each month.

THE SEX HORMONES

Both men and women produce sex hormones, but the effects are greatest in women. Sex hormones are responsible for the development of the secondary sex characteristics in both sexes and for cyclical changes in women's bodies that begin at menarche (the onset of menstruation) and cease at menopause. They also prepare and maintain pregnancies. In men, hormones control sexual development, the production of sperm and the maintenance of sex drive.

THE EFFECTS ON MEN

As a man goes through puberty, his testicles make increasing amounts of testosterone and this initiates a variety of changes — the growth of the penis, scrotum, and testicles, as well as that of pubic hair, muscles, and bones. Testosterone, like other androgens, has an anabolic effect: it raises the rate of protein synthesis and lowers the rate at which it is broken down. This increases muscle bulk, especially in the chest and shoulders, and accelerates growth. (Testosterone also promotes aggression, a characteristic male trait.)

If testosterone production becomes reduced, a man's sexual drive and performance will fall off. This can happen where there is disease or atrophy of the testes due to advanced age. (Unlike with women, a male climacteric that involves a dramatic shift in hormone balance is considered a disease.) Rather than decreasing abruptly, from the age of 40, the hormone-producing cells in the testes begin to decrease in number, so less testosterone is produced and by extreme old age, there is about a half to a third of that in younger men.

Regular sexual activity is the best way of keeping testosterone levels up while lack of sexual activity will cause it to decrease. If you don't have a partner, regular masturbation can be just as effective. If a sex drive has been depressed, it can take a couple of months to recover a normal one.

THE EFFECTS ON WOMEN

The production of ovarian and pituitary hormones affect all of the organs in a woman's body. While not all the changes are visible, those that are can easily be observed since they are pronounced. These changes can involve the mind as well as the body and can produce varying emotions. Changes due to hormones are most apparent at different stages of the menstrual cycle, during pregnancy and after childbirth, and at menopause.

THE MENSTRUAL CYCLE

The menstrual cycle begins on day one of menstruation when small quantities of estrogen are produced by the ovaries. These gradually increase until they reach a peak just prior to ovulation, which occurs 14 days after the first day of menstruation. With the emission of an ovum the remaining follicle, the corpus luteum, begins to secrete progesterone, reaching a peak a few days prior to the onset of menstruation.

The average length of the menstrual cycle is 28 days but the normal range can be anything between 26 and 33 days. The first half of the cycle, before ovulation, is termed the estrogenic phase of the cycle and the second half, after ovulation, is the progestergenic phase. During the second half of the progestergenic phase there is a small surge of estrogen secretion that dies away with the progesterone levels a few days prior to menstruation. The steeply falling levels of female hormones and final withdrawal result in the shedding of the uterine lining and the menstrual blood flow.

Bleeding occurs because the endometrial lining crumbles and falls away. In the second half of the cycle (the progestergenic phase), the lining that, under the action of progesterone, has become thick and filled with glands in preparation for receiving a fertilized egg, is shed if conception does not occur.

Menstruation, therefore, has two functions: getting rid of the old uterine lining, which is not used for a pregnancy; and preparing the body for the whole cycle to begin again in case pregnancy should occur the next month.

HORMONAL CHANGES IN THE BODY

In the first half of the menstrual cycle, estrogen production has a youthful effect on the body. It keeps the hair in good condition, it makes the skin bloom, and it raises the mood. Vaginal discharge is thin, clear, and runny with very little odor.

In the second half, progesterone shows its effects by causing the breasts to enlarge and become heavy and tender with a nodular consistency; pimples may appear, and vaginal secretions become thicker and more rubbery, and may have a fishy odor.

Other changes attributed to progesterone production include water retention, which can make a woman feel bloated with a puffy face, hands, and feet; have a thickened waistline; experience headaches and abdominal pains; and suffer enormous changes in mood such as irritability, loss of temper, tearfulness, and depression that can lead to suicidal feelings and violence.

CLIMACTERIC

The climacteric describes the period of a woman's life when ovarian function gradually wanes, and levels of estrogen and progesterone decline. During the menarche, it takes several years for regular ovarian activity and hormone production to be established. The climacteric spans a similar length of time, and menopause or cessation of menstruation is only a part of the whole syndrome.

MENOPAUSAL SYMPTOMS

Many women experience no symptoms at all during the climacteric and hardly know it is happening; others suffer very troublesome menopausal symptoms such as hot flashes, night sweats, mood changes, loss of sexual urge, and depression. Hormone replacement therapy (HRT) can treat 90 to 95 percent of these symptoms successfully.

There has been a tendency to believe that menopause ushers in a period of gradual decline into old age, but this need not be so. For an ever-increasing number of women, it is a time of great personal development, with the acquisition of new skills and newfound self-assurance.

There is no way of finding out when your own menopause will occur, but patterns tend to run in families, so women often have early or late menopauses similar to their mother's.

The age range for menopause is 40 to 56; only one percent of women have a cessation of periods at the age of 40, but by the age of 56, 99 percent of all women have gone through the climacteric.

CONTRACEPTION

There are several ways in which couples can have intercourse without a resulting pregnancy, but these vary greatly in their reliability and ease of use. In terms of effectiveness, the best solution is for either the man or the woman to have a sterilization operation. At the other end of the scale, the simplest — but most risky — form of contraception is the withdrawal method (coitus interruptus), in which the man withdraws his penis from his partner's vagina before he ejaculates.

In between these two extremes there are three other main forms of contraception: the natural or rhythm methods, mechanical (or barrier) contraception and hormonal contraception (the Pill).

NATURAL, MECHANICAL, AND HORMONAL

Natural or rhythm methods, including calendar, temperature, or cervical mucus methods, involve restricting intercourse to those days of the woman's monthly cycle when conception is unlikely. These days are determined through calculation or observation of various phenomena. Mechanical methods, such as the condom or diaphragm, create barriers that prevent the sperm from reaching the ovum, so that fertilization cannot take place, while hormonal contraception involves taking hormones that affect the metabolism and physiology of the body to prevent conception.

Mechanical methods exist for both men and women, but while hormonal methods of contraception could, in theory, be used by either sex, those inhibiting ovulation in women are the most advanced and prevalent.

Ever since the advent of hormonal contraceptives for women — the Pill, with its ease, simplicity, and almost 100 percent efficacy — contraception has largely been seen as the responsibility of women and initially, at least, women were glad to take on this responsibility because with it went greater sexual freedom.

Recently, however, mechanical contraception, in the form of condoms, has become more popular. This is partly because of fears about possible side effects of the Pill, but it is mainly because, with the increasing prevalence of herpes and AIDS (transmitted in most cases by sexual contact), the use of condoms has become associated with "safe sex." Condoms, once scorned because of their comparatively low efficacy in preventing conception compared to the Pill, are now enjoying a renaissance. This change in contraceptive preference reflects increased responsibility for preventing pregnancy on the man's part (and about time, too).

MALE CONTRACEPTION

The most ancient form of male contraception is coitus interruptus: withdrawal of the penis just prior to ejaculation. This is a dangerous and ineffective method of contraception. Prior to ejaculation there may be a preemission of a small amount of seminal fluid, and this may contain some sperm. This has resulted in many a pregnancy, and coitus interruptus should never be relied upon to prevent pregnancy, nor practiced if pregnancy is unwanted.

Vasectomy is a permanent method of birth control for men and can be done in a simple, 15-20 minute operation on an outpatient basis under local anesthetic. The sheath or condom is the most popular form of male contraceptive. It is a fairly effective method of birth control, and one of the oldest.

THE CONDOM

Made of thin rubber and placed on the erect penis prior to penetration, the condom retains the ejaculate so that sperm are prevented from entering the woman. For added protection, and to add lubrication and prevent friction, spermicidal jelly or cream should also be used. Condoms are available in different shapes, colors, thicknesses, and textures, and some are lubricated and already covered with spermicide. A condom can only be used once, so a new one is needed for each act of intercourse.

After ejaculation, the penis and condom should be withdrawn while the penis is still partially erect; the condom should be held firmly in place on the penis during withdrawal so that no semen can leak into the vagina.

There are advantages to the condom: it can be effective if used properly and with spermicidal preparations, it is readily available, easy to use, and can be worn by all men. Most importantly, it provides protection against sexually transmitted infections and may protect women from cervical cancer.

However, condoms are not universally popular. For instance, some men feel a loss of sensation when wearing a condom, although this can be a useful effect for a man who ejaculates prematurely. In addition, but very occasionally, the rubber and chemicals used to manufacture condoms can cause rare allergic reactions. But the greatest objection to the condom is that it is unaesthetic and destroys the spontaneity of sexual union.

USING CONDOMS SUCCESSFULLY

• Use a new condom for each sex act and inspect it beforehand for tears or holes.
• Make sure the condom is put on before the penis comes anywhere near the vagina.
• Withdraw the penis before erection subsides completely and hold on to the rim of the condom.
• Check carefully after use for tears.
• Do not use petroleum jelly (Vaseline) to lubricate the condom; it can rot rubber and it may be irritating to the vagina. Use water-soluble jelly (see p.244).

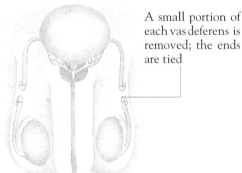

A small portion of each vas deferens is removed; the ends are tied

Vasectomy
The altered ends are tied and replaced in the scrotum. This procedure is 100 percent effective; recovery is rapid and there is no change in hormone levels or the appearance of semen. The sex drive is also unaffected.

CONTRACEPTIVE METHODS

Methods of contraception range from the simple but very risky withdrawal method to the more complicated procedure of surgical sterilization, but there are many safe, nonpermanent, and readily accessible methods of birth control available. You can buy condoms, the sponge, and spermicidal suppositories, creams, and jellies over the counter at the drugstore. The diaphragm or cap must be measured by a specialist for your exact size and changed along with gains or losses in weight or after childbirth. IUDs also must be inserted and removed by a specialist, and regularly checked by the wearer. All the types of birth control pills are available only by prescription.

Contraceptive pill
There are various forms; some contain estrogen only, some progesterone, and some a combination of both.

Condom
The primary male method, these rubber barriers come in a variety of colors, textures, and thicknesses.

Intrauterine device (IUD)
Once fitted, it remains in place for one to three years. Some versions contain copper or progesterone.

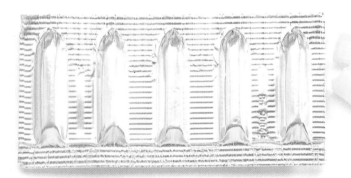

Spermicidal suppositories
These can be used alone or in combination with the condom or diaphragm. A new one should be used for each act of intercourse.

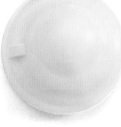

Cervical cap
Similar to though smaller than a diaphragm, it fits tightly over the cervix.

Diaphragm
One of the barrier methods, it prevents sperm from entering the uterus and is used with spermicidal cream or jelly.

Spermicidal sponge
An over-the-counter barrier method that is easy to insert and should be left in the vagina at least six hours after intercourse.

Spermicidal jellies and creams
These are used for contraceptive purposes in combination with a diaphragm or condom, and also to protect against sexually transmitted disease.

FEMALE CONTRACEPTION

The forms of contraception available to women include mechanical methods (diaphragm and cap, IUD, and female condom), hormonal methods (the combined and mini pills), tubal sterilization, and the natural methods.

THE DIAPHRAGM AND CAP

The diaphragm is a rubber dome mounted on a pliable metal rim. Before intercourse, you insert it into your vagina so that it fits behind the pubic bone and blocks the entrance to the cervix and prevents sperm from entering the uterus. Used in conjunction with chemical spermicides (which you apply to the diaphragm prior to insertion and repeat after three hours in jelly, foam, or suppository form while the diaphragm is still in place), it is a very reliable method of birth control and one that provides some protection against venereal disease.

The diaphragm is available from your doctor, and should be checked for size after a change in weight of more than 20 pounds (9 kilograms) either way, or after childbirth or a miscarriage; the vagina can change shape under these circumstances.

After removal, the diaphragm should be gently washed in warm water, rinsed, dried, and stored in a cool place. Always check your diaphragm for holes and tears, and do not remove it for six to eight hours after intercourse. The diaphragm should not be left in place in the vagina indefinitely.

A cap is similar to, and used in the same way as, a diaphragm except that it is smaller and covers just the cervix.

INTRAUTERINE DEVICES (IUDs)

These devices, known as coils or loops, are small (1-2 inch [2.5 cms]), flat, flexible objects made of plastic which are inserted by a doctor into a woman's uterus. A short, soft plastic string, attached to the IUD to enable it to be removed, protrudes from the cervix and can be felt with the fingers.

IUDs are second only to the Pill in efficacy in preventing pregnancies. They work by making the uterus hostile to the implantation of a fertilized embryo. Once inserted, they can be left in place for a year or more. The new designs of IUDs can be worn by all women, including those who have not had a baby.

One of the advantages of IUDs is that once inserted, they provide immediate and continued protection and do not interrupt lovemaking. Unlike the Pill, they do not interfere with breast milk production or natural hormone balance, and they do not interfere with a woman's natural fertility.

IUDs, however, can cause pelvic inflammatory disease and, as a result, are no longer widely recommended.

FEMALE CONDOMS

Although not a new idea (they were available back in the 1920s, but never caught on), female condoms are being hailed as the latest in contraception for women. Still being perfected, the female condom is a thin but tough latex tube, open at one end and closed at the other and with a flexible ring at each end to make it easy to handle and to keep it in place.

Before intercourse, it is inserted into the vagina (closed end first) to create a soft, flexible lining that, like a male condom, retains the ejaculate and prevents sperm from entering the woman's body. It also provides a good measure of protection against sexually transmitted diseases.

THE COMBINED PILL

The most effective reversible method of contraception is a pill containing synthetic estrogen and progestin, hormones similar to those produced naturally by the ovaries. They alter the body's hormonal balance so that the ovaries cease to ovulate and pregnancy is prevented. A course of pills is usually taken for 21 or 28 days and menstruation occurs after cessation of taking the pills every 28th day. Birth control pills can only be prescribed by a doctor after a thorough gynecological checkup including breast examination and a Pap smear.

They should not be taken by women who smoke, who are obese or who have a past history of clotting disorder or heart disease, or where there is a family history of heart disease. Women using the Pill should have regular checkups, take the Pill with the least amount of estrogen possible, and report any side effects — for example, visual defects, sudden onset of headaches, chest pain, pains in the legs, breathlessness, palpitations, or irregular bleeding — to their doctors.

MINI PILLS

Mini pills rely on progestin for their contraceptive effect and contain no estrogen. They have fewer side effects than the combined pill, but while the combined pill totally suppresses ovulation, mini pills do not, so that menstruation is determined by your own internal cycle. In some women this results in a rather irregular menstrual pattern.

Mini pills prevent conception by partially suppressing ovulation and additionally by interfering with the cervix, uterus, and Fallopian tubes, making them hostile to sperm and implantation. The mini pill is usually taken daily on a continuous basis, and may be a better solution than the combined pill for women who are concerned about taking large amounts of estrogen.

Norplant, a progestin delivery system, works like the mini pill, but offers long-term contraception. A doctor makes an incision in the woman's arm and inserts five small tubes; these remain in place for up to five years. When the woman wants to restore fertility, Norplant is

removed under local anesthetic. The product's effectiveness is similar to that of the mini pill.

TUBAL STERILIZATION

This method of contraception should only be considered by women who no longer want to bear children, because it should be seen as permanent. There are five different operations available, in which the tubes can be tied, clipped, sutured, or cauterized, thereby blocking them and preventing an ovum and sperm ever meeting. All the methods involve tying or closing the tubes, but a portion of the tubes is invariably removed. This operation is therefore almost impossible to reverse. There is a very low failure rate with this operation — about four in every 1,000 — and serious complications from tubal sterilization are rare.

NATURAL OR RHYTHM METHODS

Three birth control methods based on natural body cycles — enabling couples to avoid having intercourse on those days when conception is most likely — have proved partially effective under ideal conditions.

The first, the calendar method, uses the onset of bleeding as day one and interprets the four days on either side of day 14 as the fertile period, during which time intercourse has to be avoided to prevent conception.

The temperature method relies on recording the body temperature daily on a chart and noting when the temperature remains elevated for three days. During the period of elevation and just before it, intercourse should be avoided; this is the fertile time.

The cervical mucus method involves observing the normal changes in vaginal discharge so that you can predict ovulation and the days unsafe for intercourse.

Of course, all these methods are without medical risk — the most common side effect is pregnancy. They do; however, interfere substantially with the frequency of intercourse.

MAN: DO YOU HAVE A MEDICAL PROBLEM?

HAVE ONE OR BOTH TESTES SUDDENLY BECOME PAINFUL?

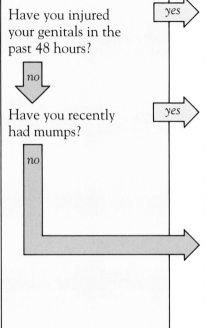

Have you injured your genitals in the past 48 hours? — *yes*

Internal damage to the testes as a result of injury may have caused the pain, especially if there is also swelling. Call your doctor now. You may need to spend some time in the hospital, where your problem can be treated surgically.

no

Have you recently had mumps? — *yes*

Orchitis, a fairly common swelling of one or both testes, is probably the cause. In rare cases, the disorder may result in infertility. Consult your doctor, who will examine you to rule out the possibility of your having a more serious infection of the lymph glands. The doctor will probably prescribe painkillers for you to take to relieve the pain and advise you to rest in bed.

no

Torsion of the testes (twisting of the testes inside the scrotum) is possible. This can happen at any time, even during sleep, and may be accompanied by nausea and vomiting. Get medical help now.

HAVE ONE OR BOTH TESTES BECOME SWOLLEN?

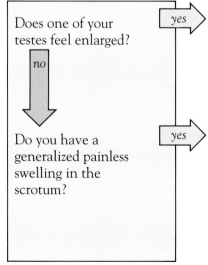

Does one of your testes feel enlarged? — *yes*

A cyst (fluid-filled sac) may have formed inside the scrotum. Although such cysts are harmless and can grow quite large before causing any discomfort, it is nevertheless important to see your doctor so that he or she can rule out the possibility of a tumor. Cysts are most common in men over the age of 40, although they can occur at any age.

no

Do you have a generalized painless swelling in the scrotum? — *yes*

Hydrocele, an accumulation of a clear, thin fluid between the fibrous layers that cover the testes, is possible. You may need to have the fluid drawn off by needle under local anesthetic. If the problem recurs, your doctor may advise you to have a minor operation to tighten or remove one of the fibrous layers so that the fluid can no longer accumulate.

IS YOUR PENIS SORE?

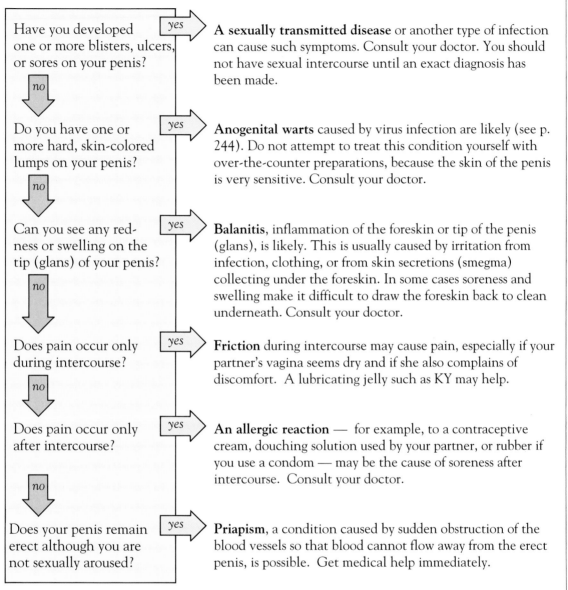

Have you developed one or more blisters, ulcers, or sores on your penis?

yes → **A sexually transmitted disease** or another type of infection can cause such symptoms. Consult your doctor. You should not have sexual intercourse until an exact diagnosis has been made.

no ↓

Do you have one or more hard, skin-colored lumps on your penis?

yes → **Anogenital warts** caused by virus infection are likely (see p. 244). Do not attempt to treat this condition yourself with over-the-counter preparations, because the skin of the penis is very sensitive. Consult your doctor.

no ↓

Can you see any redness or swelling on the tip (glans) of your penis?

yes → **Balanitis**, inflammation of the foreskin or tip of the penis (glans), is likely. This is usually caused by irritation from infection, clothing, or from skin secretions (smegma) collecting under the foreskin. In some cases soreness and swelling make it difficult to draw the foreskin back to clean underneath. Consult your doctor.

no ↓

Does pain occur only during intercourse?

yes → **Friction** during intercourse may cause pain, especially if your partner's vagina seems dry and if she also complains of discomfort. A lubricating jelly such as KY may help.

no ↓

Does pain occur only after intercourse?

yes → **An allergic reaction** — for example, to a contraceptive cream, douching solution used by your partner, or rubber if you use a condom — may be the cause of soreness after intercourse. Consult your doctor.

no ↓

Does your penis remain erect although you are not sexually aroused?

yes → **Priapism**, a condition caused by sudden obstruction of the blood vessels so that blood cannot flow away from the erect penis, is possible. Get medical help immediately.

BLOOD IN THE SEMEN

Pinkish, reddish, or brownish streaks in your semen, hemospermia, may be caused by the presence of blood. Uncommonly, small veins in the upper part of the urethra may rupture during an erection. These heal themselves within a few minutes, although the semen may continue to be slightly discolored for a few days afterward. This is usually no cause for concern, but you should consult your doctor if you are worried.

WOMAN: DO YOU HAVE A MEDICAL PROBLEM?

HAVE YOU NOTICED A VAGINAL DISCHARGE THAT IS UNUSUAL IN COLOR OR CONSISTENCY?

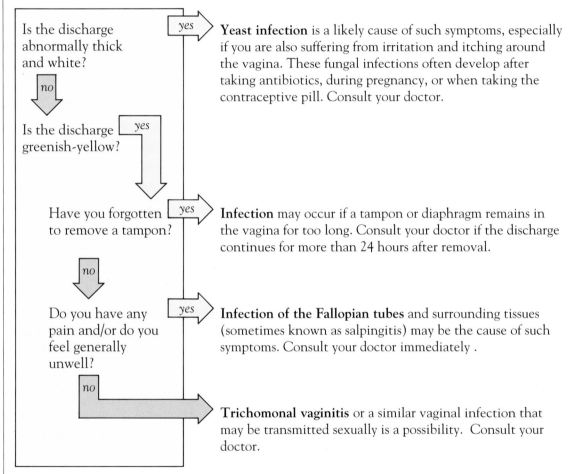

Is the discharge abnormally thick and white?

yes

Yeast infection is a likely cause of such symptoms, especially if you are also suffering from irritation and itching around the vagina. These fungal infections often develop after taking antibiotics, during pregnancy, or when taking the contraceptive pill. Consult your doctor.

no

Is the discharge greenish-yellow?

yes

Have you forgotten to remove a tampon?

yes

Infection may occur if a tampon or diaphragm remains in the vagina for too long. Consult your doctor if the discharge continues for more than 24 hours after removal.

no

Do you have any pain and/or do you feel generally unwell?

yes

Infection of the Fallopian tubes and surrounding tissues (sometimes known as salpingitis) may be the cause of such symptoms. Consult your doctor immediately .

no

Trichomonal vaginitis or a similar vaginal infection that may be transmitted sexually is a possibility. Consult your doctor.

BLOOD IN THE URINE

Small amounts of cloudy, bloodstained, and/ or strong-smelling urine passed more frequently than usual may be the result of cystitis (inflammation of the bladder) or urethritis (inflammation of the urethra).

You should consult your doctor, who, if you have an infection, probably will prescribe antibiotics and medicine to make your urine less acid.

DO YOU BLEED BETWEEN PERIODS OR, IF YOU ARE POSTMENOPAUSAL, AFTER THE CESSATION OF PERIODS?

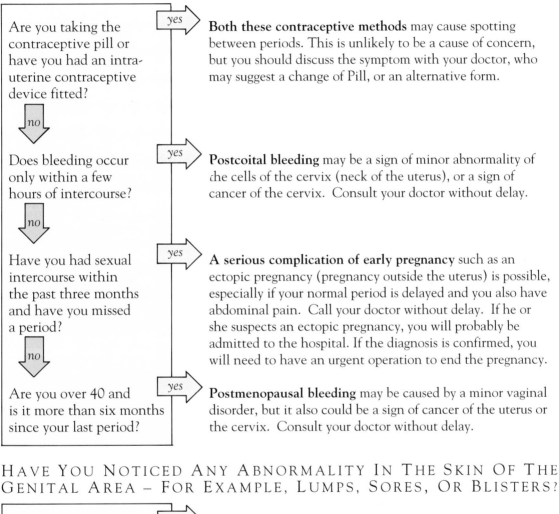

Are you taking the contraceptive pill or have you had an intra-uterine contraceptive device fitted?

yes → **Both these contraceptive methods** may cause spotting between periods. This is unlikely to be a cause of concern, but you should discuss the symptom with your doctor, who may suggest a change of Pill, or an alternative form.

no

Does bleeding occur only within a few hours of intercourse?

yes → **Postcoital bleeding** may be a sign of minor abnormality of the cells of the cervix (neck of the uterus), or a sign of cancer of the cervix. Consult your doctor without delay.

no

Have you had sexual intercourse within the past three months and have you missed a period?

yes → **A serious complication of early pregnancy** such as an ectopic pregnancy (pregnancy outside the uterus) is possible, especially if your normal period is delayed and you also have abdominal pain. Call your doctor without delay. If he or she suspects an ectopic pregnancy, you will probably be admitted to the hospital. If the diagnosis is confirmed, you will need to have an urgent operation to end the pregnancy.

no

Are you over 40 and is it more than six months since your last period?

yes → **Postmenopausal bleeding** may be caused by a minor vaginal disorder, but it also could be a sign of cancer of the uterus or the cervix. Consult your doctor without delay.

HAVE YOU NOTICED ANY ABNORMALITY IN THE SKIN OF THE GENITAL AREA – FOR EXAMPLE, LUMPS, SORES, OR BLISTERS?

Do you use soap, bath salts, or deodorants in the genital area and/or vaginal douches?

yes → **Irritation from perfumes and chemicals** in any of these may cause inflammation of the delicate skin of the vulva and the sensitive lining of the vagina. Avoid excessive use of soap in the genital area — plain water is best.

no → **A skin condition affecting the vulva** is likely to be the cause of the irritation. Consult your doctor for a firm diagnosis and treatment.

DO YOU FEEL PAIN DURING INTERCOURSE?

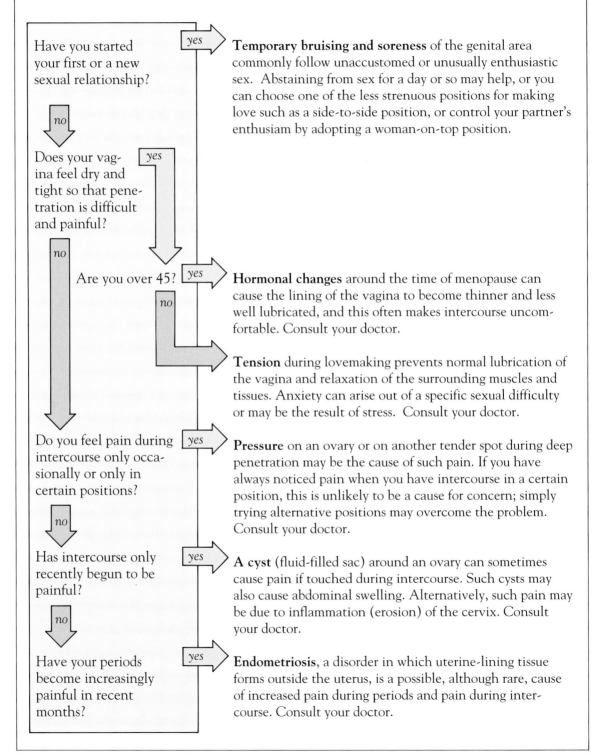

Have you started your first or a new sexual relationship? — *yes* →

Temporary bruising and soreness of the genital area commonly follow unaccustomed or unusually enthusiastic sex. Abstaining from sex for a day or so may help, or you can choose one of the less strenuous positions for making love such as a side-to-side position, or control your partner's enthusiam by adopting a woman-on-top position.

no ↓

Does your vagina feel dry and tight so that penetration is difficult and painful? — *yes* →

no ↓

Are you over 45? — *yes* →

Hormonal changes around the time of menopause can cause the lining of the vagina to become thinner and less well lubricated, and this often makes intercourse uncomfortable. Consult your doctor.

no →

Tension during lovemaking prevents normal lubrication of the vagina and relaxation of the surrounding muscles and tissues. Anxiety can arise out of a specific sexual difficulty or may be the result of stress. Consult your doctor.

Do you feel pain during intercourse only occasionally or only in certain positions? — *yes* →

Pressure on an ovary or on another tender spot during deep penetration may be the cause of such pain. If you have always noticed pain when you have intercourse in a certain position, this is unlikely to be a cause for concern; simply trying alternative positions may overcome the problem. Consult your doctor.

no ↓

Has intercourse only recently begun to be painful? — *yes* →

A cyst (fluid-filled sac) around an ovary can sometimes cause pain if touched during intercourse. Such cysts may also cause abdominal swelling. Alternatively, such pain may be due to inflammation (erosion) of the cervix. Consult your doctor.

no ↓

Have your periods become increasingly painful in recent months? — *yes* →

Endometriosis, a disorder in which uterine-lining tissue forms outside the uterus, is a possible, although rare, cause of increased pain during periods and pain during intercourse. Consult your doctor.

SEXUALLY TRANSMITTED DISEASES

STDs are those contracted during sexual contact, be it oral, genital, or anal. To a degree, sexually transmitted diseases can be divided into ancient and modern. The older sexually transmitted diseases include gonorrhea, syphilis, urethritis, trichomoniasis, yeast infections, and pubic lice. The most serious, as well as the most modern, are AIDS, genital herpes, and chlamydia.

Two or three centuries ago, syphilis was the scourge of many continents, killing hundreds of thousands of people. Nowadays, gonorrhea and syphilis can be treated simply and completely cured with antibiotics such as penicillin. Pubic lice ("crabs") can be eradicated with a special shampoo in the same way as head lice, and trichomoniasis and yeast infections are amenable to powerful specific therapies which get rid of them in one short course.

THE HOW AND WHY OF TREATMENT

Some of the sexually transmitted diseases, however (particularly chlamydia), can be difficult to treat because they are symptomless. In women, a pelvic examination will not give a reliable diagnosis of chlamydia; successful diagnosis depends on the laboratory culture of vaginal secretions. The absence of symptoms means that such an infection can take a strong hold and make treatment difficult once it has begun. More importantly, it means that a carrier can unwittingly spread the disease to any number of people, depending on how promiscuous his or her sexual behavior.

The nearest source of specialist advice and treatment for sexually transmitted disease is the local family planning clinic. Many clinics have a resident counselor who can advise you about treatment, a change in lifestyle, and coming to terms with the fact that you have a sexually transmitted disease. The importance of contacting all your sexual partners is stressed and you should be cooperative in helping the clinic to track down these people.

The advent of AIDS has certainly led to a more responsible attitude to sex in the community at large. Statisticians now say that people are taking fewer sexual partners than before, resulting in a 70 percent decrease in sexually transmitted diseases. More and more people are practicing safe sex by using condoms (see p.244) and the more people who take up this practice, the more rapid will be the downward trend in the numbers of people suffering from sexually transmitted diseases.

VAGINAL INFECTIONS

Chlamydia, yeast infections, and trichomoniasis are all vaginal infections, but they can infect men as well as women. Of the three, chlamydia is by far the most worrying because its presence is not always obvious and, if left untreated, it can lead to more serious infections.

CHLAMYDIA

Chlamydia is rapidly becoming the most common sexually transmitted disease. It is also the greatest problem because most women affected with chlamydia will have no symptoms. The side effects of the infection are extremely serious, however, and so anyone who suspects that they have an infection should go to a doctor immediately to have it correctly diagnosed.

Chlamydia may damage the lining of the vagina, mouth, eyes, urinary tract, and rectum, although it is usually confined to the cervix, leading to an offensive, yellow-colored discharge. The most worrisome aspect of this infection is that 30 percent of all cases may develop into a generalized pelvic infection that can result in infertility due to a blockage of the tubes by scarring. A woman who is infected may pass on the infection to her baby during childbirth; the commonest symptom of chlamydia in newborns is conjunctivitis, but it can occasionally cause pneumonia.

The symptoms of chlamydia are usually sparse, but any unusual cervical discharge should alert a woman to its possibility. There may be occasional fever and abdominal discomfort, particularly with intercourse, and male partners may have urinary problems, experiencing pain when passing urine.

Chlamydia is very easy to treat once the diagnosis has been made with the modern tests available. A specimen of vaginal discharge will yield a diagnosis within 30-60 minutes, permitting immediate treatment.

Chlamydia is completely curable with a course of antibiotics, but the medication must be taken exactly as prescribed, and the full course completed. It is dangerous to stop taking the medication if the symptoms disappear because the infection could return, and the medicines become less effective.

Any sexually active person runs the risk of catching chlamydia, but people with multiple partners run the greatest risk. If you have many sexual contacts and you contract chlamydia, all of them must be informed of the infection and be screened and treated as necessary. Re-infection can be prevented by using barrier contraceptives such as condoms and diaphragms with spermicidal creams.

YEAST INFECTIONS

Yeast infections are caused by the fungus (yeast) organisms monilia and candida. Monilia is a normal resident of the vagina, and infection occurs when it is allowed to overgrow. This may come about if vaginal douches are used or antiseptics are put in the bath water, since these suppress the normal flora which keep the growth under control. These infections are more common in certain groups of women, which include:

• Women taking antibiotics: the number of fungi in the vagina is normally kept in check by bacteria that also live there. If an antibiotic kills these bacteria, the fungi can overgrow.

• Women with diabetes. When diabetes becomes unstable, the presence of sugar in the urine provides a favorable medium for all organisms, and monilia can get out of hand like the rest.

• Women taking synthetic progesterones, the most common example being the contraceptive pill which, containing a high dose of progesterone, encourages the growth of candida.

• Women with their own high progesterone levels, for example premenstrual women and pregnant women.

The symptoms of yeast infections are a thick, white, curdy vaginal discharge with soreness, irritation, and itching of the vagina and perineum. Quite often, the skin becomes red and scaly and the rash may spread to the inner sides of the thighs. A man who contracts the infection from a woman will have this red, scaly, itchy rash on the penis, the scrotum, the skin of the genital area, and down the side of the thighs. In both men and women, if the infection ascends the rectum there will be soreness, itching, and even diarrhea.

If you get a yeast infection, refrain from intercourse until the infection is cleared. Consult your doctor and get a complete course of treatment; this may be for seven days and may be in the form of suppositories or cream. In some severe cases you may have to take therapy in three forms: a cream to be applied to the skin; suppositories to be used in the vagina; and lozenges to be taken by mouth to clear the gut of excessive yeast organisms.

Do not scratch the affected areas, because the fungus can get under your nails and you will spread it. Preparations for the treatment of vaginal yeast infections are available over-the-counter; if you have had a yeast infection treated in the past and the symptoms recur, you may now be able to buy the same product at a pharmacy.

TRICHOMONIASIS

Trichomoniasis is a disease that affects both men and women. The organism lives in the vagina, cervix, urethra, and bladder of women and in the urethra and prostate of men. It is most common in sexually active women and 90 percent of their partners are infected, too. Men have few symptoms other than, occasionally, a discharge from the penis and a burning sensation on passing urine. Women have an offensive yellow vaginal discharge, soreness and itching of the vagina and perineum, and burning with passing urine. If the infection affects the bladder, there may be symptoms of cystitis, with frequency, urgency, burning, and pain at the end of urination.

Both partners and all their other sexual contacts must be treated. The disease is treated with a drug called Flagyl, taken by mouth as a single eight-tablet dose or as a seven-day course of one tablet three times a day. The Flagyl should be taken with meals to minimize gastric upset, and you may experience side effects such as a strange taste in your mouth and a furry coating on your tongue. While you are on a course of Flagyl, you should avoid alcohol since you may get abdominal pain. Do not take Flagyl for longer than a week at a time, and do not take it at all if you are pregnant. If you need a second course, ask for a blood count as Flagyl may occasionally affect blood cell production. Douches, creams, and pessaries should never be relied on as treatments for trichomoniasis.

AVOIDING VAGINAL INFECTIONS

All vaginal infections are more common during periods of stress when a woman's general physical condition is poor. Being overweight may also make you more prone to infection because the folds of fat may cause collections of vaginal secretions and sweat. Having a new sexual partner, or having several, is also associated with the increase of likelihood of vaginal infections.

• Using a condom is the best protection against vaginal infections, not only with a new partner but when you have more than one partner, especially if you are being reinfected by your regular partner.

• Practice good vaginal hygiene by keeping the area clean and dry.

• Bathe carefully, wipe from front to back, and avoid douches, hygiene sprays, bubble baths, and bath oils.

• If you need extra lubrication during intercourse, use a contraceptive foam or a cream or a jelly which offers some protection against infection. Never use petroleum jelly (such as Vaseline); it is hard to remove and it might promote infection.

• Wear cotton underpants and avoid nylon pants, panty hose and tight slacks, which hold moisture in the vaginal area.

NSU, Gonorrhea, And Syphilis

NSU (Nonspecific Urethritis) is one of the commonest sexually transmitted diseases; one person in 500 catches it. Gonorrhea and syphilis, once very common, are now much less of a problem in terms of the number of people they affect.

NSU

The causes of NSU are not known with any certainty, but one of the chief culprits is probably the organism responsible for chlamydia (see p.236). The symptoms develop about a week to ten days after intercourse with an infected person, although NSU can also appear without any sexual contact, and treatment consists of a long course of antibiotics.

Eighty percent of the sufferers are men. Their first noticeable symptom is a slight tingling at the tip of the penis — sometimes felt when urinating the first thing in the morning. A scanty, clear discharge may be present. This discharge becomes thicker over time if the condition remains untreated. Eventually the symptoms fade, but the infection may remain dormant and can still be transmitted. NSU may be symptomless in women, or there may be a slight increase in vaginal discharge. Because it may not be noticed, it is vital that if a man contracts NSU, his partner or partners should also be treated.

Gonorrhea

Gonorrhea (or "clap") is caused by a bacterium, neisseria gonorrhoeae, and although it affects both men and women, it causes symptoms primarily in men. In women, the disease may be symptomless and therefore more dangerous, because a woman may be infected without knowing it and so will not seek diagnosis and treatment. This can lead to chronic inflammation in the pelvis, and if the ovaries and Fallopian tubes are affected, scarring may cause sterility. In addition, a mother who is incubating gonorrhea may pass on the infection to her newborn baby during labor, and the baby will develop a serious form of conjunctivitis.

Gonorrhea In Men

The commonest symptom of gonorrhea in men is a yellow, offensive discharge from the penis, and there may also be sores around the genitals. If gonorrhea remains untreated, it can spread to the vas deferens and cause sterility, and may also lead to arthritis. Any man who experiences such symptoms, and any woman who has had sex with a man who has any kind of discharge from the penis, should seek help from a family planning clinic or a doctor as soon as possible.

Gonorrhea In Women

An infected woman, if she shows any symptoms, may have a discharge from the urethra, but more often there will be a vaginal discharge with pain and burning when passing urine. With a severe infection that ascends to the bladder, there may be cystitis and the presence of blood in the urine. Not surprisingly, the entire perineum may be sore and inflamed and if the rectum is involved there will be pain when passing stools. If the couple has engaged in oral sex, the bacterium may cause soreness and inflammation of the throat.

The diagnosis of gonorrhea in a woman is not easy and relies on special swabs being taken from the urethra, the cervix, and the rectum. Laboratory examination of the swabs can give the results within 24 hours. Always go to a doctor and ask for these tests to be done if you have any suspicion that your partner has a venereal disease, and avoid any sexual contact with anyone until you have been diagnosed, fully treated, and declared free of the disease. You should be suspicious if any sexual partner has a discharge from his penis, if there are any sores around his genitals, or if you develop a sore in your own genital area within a few days of sexual contact.

TREATMENT   The incidence of gonorrhea has been greatly reduced since the advent of the newer penicillins, which are the mainstay of treatment for both men and women. They can be given in a slow-release, injectable form which requires only one injection, making treatment quick and immediate. Occasionally, a penicillin-resistant strain of the bacterium will need treatment with tetracycline given in tablet form over a four-day period.

At the end of treatment, a woman should have a gynecological examination to make sure that there is no inflammation in the pelvis and should have repeat swabs done to make sure that all the bacteria have been eradicated.

Gonorrhea is most common in people under the age of 25 who have many sexual partners. If you fit into this category you should have a check-up every six months, and use condoms to decrease the probability of your getting an infection or being reinfected. If any of your symptoms persist, you may have become reinfected. Make sure that your partner seeks medical attention and full treatment if he or she is a carrier of the disease.

SYPHILIS

Syphilis ("pox") is caused by a spirochete (spiral-shaped) bacterium, treponema pallidum. Two or three centuries ago it spread throughout Europe like wildfire, killing hundreds of thousands of people in widespread epidemics, but today it is far less common.

It affects the skin, the internal organs, and eventually the brain and nerves, causing paralysis, insanity, and finally death. In the course of its development it may mimic any number of other diseases, causing swollen joints, spinal pain, deformities, and heart disease. When it was widespread, syphilis was called the great imitator and in some ways AIDS is its latter-day successor. However, the syphilis bacterium succumbs very quickly to penicillin and the disease is almost a thing of the past.

It is transmitted by sexual contact from open sores called chancres (pronounced "shankers") which are found on the genital organs, the mouth, and the skin of the genital area where the bacterium has penetrated the skin, so they are not uncommon on the edge of the vagina, the vulva, and the cervix. They are hardened, red-rimmed, painless pimples.

Syphilis has three stages, and the first two are highly infectious. Primary syphilis (the first stage) occurs about three weeks after sexual contact with an infected person, and the onset of symptoms — the appearance of one or more chancres — can occur anywhere from nine to 90 days later. The chancre will disappear within two to six weeks, even without treatment, and only a small percentage of women who develop a chancre will notice it because it is often hidden deep within the vagina.

The second stage, secondary syphilis, occurs anywhere from one week to six months after the initial chancre heals. Symptoms include a rash, fever, sore throat, headaches, loss of appetite, nausea, inflamed eyes, and loss of hair. This stage can last anywhere from three to six months or even several years.

Tertiary syphilis, the third and final stage, may appear in ten to 20 years and can result in heart disease, brain damage, spinal cord damage, and blindness. About one in every four people not treated in the secondary stage will eventually die or will be incapacitated from syphilis.

TREATMENT   Penicillin or tetracyclines are used for treatment and both partners must be treated at the same time or reinfection is likely. Regular blood tests will be arranged for two years after treatment to make sure there is no relapse. If it is cured in the primary and secondary stages permanent damage will be prevented. Since syphilis can be passed on to, and has dire consequences for, a developing fetus, all pregnant women should be given a blood test for it within the first four months of pregnancy and treated as necessary.

GENITAL HERPES

Genital herpes is an infectious, recurring disease caused mainly by the virus herpes simplex II, a close relative of herpes simplex I, which causes cold sores around the mouth and face. Herpes simplex II causes 90 percent of all herpes infections of the genital area, while herpes simplex I is responsible for the remaining ten percent.

TRANSMISSION   The virus is passed on during sexual intercourse at times when it is active, causing blisters or lesions in the surface layers of the skin of the infected partner's genital area. At other times, when the virus is lying dormant within the infected person's body and causing no active symptoms, it cannot be passed on to anyone else.

It is transmitted through exposed raw areas of skin and is more common in women than in men because their genital areas are warmer and moister than men's. The disease can also be spread by contact with other parts of the body, especially the fingers, eyes, and mouth.

Herpes is a highly contagious infection. If either partner has an active blister, there is a 90 percent chance of the other one catching the disease. It is also incurable; once the virus is in the body it stays there, although current treatment can help to clear the symptoms or to suppress active bouts.

SYMPTOMS   The condition follows a naturally waxing and waning course. It causes profound physical pain in the early stages when the blisters are developing, and psychological misery as well. A sufferer is often depressed and anxious about loss of control over his or her body and is concerned about whether he or she has transmitted the disease to another person. A sufferer may also feel intense anger or outrage toward the person who passed the disease on to them.

After sexual contact with someone who has active herpes, the symptoms may appear between three and 20 days later. The condition starts with pins and needles and increased sensitivity to touch over the area of skin where the virus is becoming active. Men have an itchy feeling on the shaft of the penis; women have this feeling in their vaginal area. After a few hours, small vesicles appear in the skin which enlarge and become fluid-filled blisters.

A day or so later these blisters burst and scab over. There is severe pain accompanying the formation of blisters and the sores can remain painful for anything up to ten days. Unless the infection is aborted within the first 24 hours, it can take anything up to 14 days to clear completely and for the skin to be normal again.

TREATMENT   Until the advent of Zovirax (acyclovir), a very potent and effective antiviral agent, in 1979, there were few drugs that could treat any virus with success. Zovirax is available by prescription in ointment, cream, or tablet form, and is effective in limiting the blisters and shortening the attack if applied early enough or if tablets are taken at the onset of symptoms. Antiviral drugs like acyclovir and immunovir work by inhibiting DNA replication of the herpes simplex virus and thus arresting the spread of the disease. However, these drugs do not eliminate the virus and are methods of controlling, rather than curing, the attacks. Zovirax is an extremely expensive drug and at the present time cannot be given for long periods because long-term safety studies have not been completed. Possible side effects include nausea, vomiting, diarrhea, nervousness, depression, and joint and muscle pain.

Of the longer-established medications for herpes, idoxuridine in an ointment, liquid, or cream is still successful with some sufferers as long as it is used as soon as the tingling sensation starts. Unfortunately, none of the older medications help to prevent a recurrence of the virus. Older remedies such as daily douches with povidone-iodine solution have now largely been superseded. Herpes lesions can become infected by bacteria, and then topical or oral antibiotics may be used to treat the outbreaks.

In addition to using medication, soaking in a tepid bath or applying cold packs can soothe the pain when the blisters have ruptured.

Because there is an association between genital herpes and cervical cancer, women who have had herpes outbreaks should have cervical smear tests annually.

LIVING WITH HERPES   Because genital herpes took the world by surprise when it first became widespread about 20 years ago, it was at first considered a scourge. Now that we know something about the condition and have methods for treating it and controlling it, we know that having herpes is not the catastrophe that some people first thought it would be. For instance:

• Not all people have recurrences. Some have a few, but some may have only one after the initial attack.

• The initial attack is normally the most severe; subsequent recurrences are usually milder.

• Recurrences do not depend on having intercourse with an infected partner, and intercourse does not trigger an attack.

• When the virus is dormant between attacks, intercourse with adequate lubrication to protect you from too much friction is perfectly safe and enjoyable. The use of a condom can also protect you from excess rubbing.

• If you are prepared to recognize the early-warning symptoms and apply the medication that works for you as soon as possible, your attack may be aborted completely.

• If you have genital herpes and there are blisters present, you should act responsibly and not have sex with anybody else. After the blisters subside, you should still use a condom during sex for about four weeks.

• It is known that stress may bring on an attack, as does hard work, worry, and sleeplessness. Try to arrange your life so that stress is minimized and learn to manage your stress with relaxation exercises.

• Plenty of rest, and a balanced diet with nutritious foods such as fresh fruit and vegetables, and plenty of liquids, will help to keep attacks at bay.

• Learn to come to terms with the fact that you have the disease, and try to overcome any initial feelings you may have of being unclean, unwanted, or stigmatized. Such feelings, while perfectly understandable, are unjustified and unfair to you. If you join a self-help group or try counseling, you will begin to feel in control of your body and you will find also that the attacks become less frequent once you have reached this state of acceptance, and are under less stress.

• Remember that the virus is able to lie dormant for a number of years, and can resurface at any time. When it does, try not to feel resentful or angry or let it otherwise threaten a happy long-term relationship.

AIDS

The Human Immunodeficiency Virus (HIV) causes the body to lose its immunity to disease. Once inside the body, the virus penetrates and multiplies inside the T4 white blood cells, which play a vital part in the body's defenses against some infections and cancers. Eventually the cells burst, releasing HIV particles into the blood, which can then infect more T4 blood cells. When that happens, the body is vulnerable to attack by "opportunistic" diseases, such as certain pneumonias and cancers, that take advantage of its weakened defenses and are all too often fatal. Infection with HIV does not lead immediately to the development of AIDS; that can take as long as eight years, and so people who have HIV may not know it for some time, during which they may unwittingly pass it on to other people.

The usual test for HIV infection involves analyzing a blood sample for signs of HIV antibodies. Antibodies are substances produced by the body in response to infection by a particular virus, and the presence of HIV antibodies in a person's blood indicates that he or she has been infected by that virus. A person whose blood contains HIV antibodies is said to be "HIV positive." If you are worried that you may have been exposed to infection with HIV, contact your doctor or a clinic to arrange for a blood test. However, because there is a variable incubation period of several months between the actual time of exposure and when the victim becomes HIV positive, AIDS tests can appear negative even though the person has been infected by the virus. This is why no blood transfusion is 100 percent safe.

TRANSMISSION The main route of infection by the virus is sexual contact, because the virus is present in very large numbers in the semen of infected men. It can therefore be passed through sexual intercourse, either vaginal or anal. The virus is also present in the blood of infected people, and so it can be passed on by infected drug addicts sharing hypodermic needles with uninfected friends. It has also been transferred to hemophiliacs by contaminated blood or blood product transfusions, and an HIV-positive mother can infect her baby, either in the uterus or at the time of birth.

In theory, the transmission of the virus from one person to another during intercourse could be blocked by any physical barrier which prevents the mixing of blood, seminal fluid, and female secretions. It is now accepted that the condom provides a way of having "safe sex," as research has shown that the virus is unable to permeate any of the commercially available brands. Spermicidal preparations help, too. Something as simple as wearing condoms and using spermicides could be of enormous importance in controlling the spread of AIDS.

AIDS affects both heterosexuals and homosexuals, although at present most people with AIDS are men, because initially it was almost totally confined to the homosexual community. While homosexual men still account for the largest proportion of people infected, they have responded with alacrity to the dictates of safe sex. Now the greatest threat from AIDS is to intravenous drug users and heterosexuals.

Many tragic cases of AIDS among women have borne out the theory that only one sexual contact with an infected person is enough for someone to contract HIV. There are many recorded cases of women contracting HIV by having a single sexual contact with a man who, unknown to them, was a drug addict, sharing equipment with others. Similarly, a married woman may be infected by her husband if he has caught the virus through having affairs, homosexual or otherwise.

PROTECTING AGAINST AIDS There is a growing belief that people should be assertive in protecting themselves from AIDS. An American doctor, Helen Kaplan, urges couples to take an HIV antibody test before engaging in what she calls "wet sex" — any practice, such as vaginal intercourse without using a condom, which involves the exchange of body fluids.

Because it takes the body as long as six months after the exposure to the virus to develop antibodies, couples are advised to abstain from wet sex during this "window of infection" and then be tested a second time.

During this time, Dr. Kaplan recommends a wide spectrum of sexual activities, excluding intercourse but including sensual massage, the use of vibrators, erotic films, fantasies, rhythmic rubbing against each other's bodies while clothed, and mutual masturbation.

As many people thoroughly enjoy extended foreplay, and may not have experienced it since the heavy petting days of their youth, for them this kind of sex could be as enjoyable as full intercourse. If a man is to proceed to penetration he should wear a condom, and follow the other guidelines of safe sex.

Just as many men as women are worried about AIDS and will be grateful if the woman raises the subject, as long as it is done tactfully and not accusingly.

SYMPTOMS Some people infected with the HIV virus do not develop symptoms, though they still can infect others. A few people develop a glandular feverlike illness soon after infection, which clears up without treatment, but most feel perfectly well.

People who have had the infection for some months or years may develop permanently swollen lymph glands, and tend to develop common skin infections. Afterwards, a variety of symptoms, including fever, weight loss, and diarrhea, known as the AIDS-related complex, may develop.

TREATMENT The possibility of finding a cure for those who are already infected with HIV, and of finding a vaccine to prevent anyone else from becoming infected, is purely conjecture at the present. Most authorities believe that neither of these things will come about within the next five years. A vaccine against a virus infection works by stimulating the body's immune system to produce antibodies that will destroy that particular virus or render it harmless. It is infinitely more difficult to produce a vaccine against HIV than other viruses, because HIV acts by destroying the body's immune system, which produces the antibodies in the first place. It also mutates rapidly, changing in subtle ways that make it impossible for the antibodies to deal with it effectively.

At the present time, there is no known cure for any disease caused by a virus, although drugs such as zidovudine (AZT) may have a restraining effect on HIV and therefore prolong the lives of people with AIDS. They do not cure the disease completely, however. The only course of action to take is to treat the symptoms and the secondary illnesses that result from the weakening of the immune system.

OUTLOOK Serious infections are the most common consequences of all immune-deficiency disorders. These complications, under the heading AIDS-related complex (ARC), can cause diarrhea, weight loss, and persistent infections. ARC symptoms are treated with a variety of antibiotics, antibacterial drugs, antiviral drugs such as AZT, and antifungal drugs. The skin cancers that result from AIDS cannot, however, be treated with the usual cancer therapy; such procedures depress the immune system further.

Most people with full-blown AIDS die within two years of the disease developing. No one actually dies of AIDS itself, however; death is nearly always from an unusual form of pneumonia which hardly ever affects the general population — pneumocystis carinii — or a virulent skin cancer called Kaposi's sarcoma.

Other opportunistic infections, which under normal circumstances the body would be strong enough to fight off with ease, may be fatal in sufferers. Most recently, it has been found that the virus can affect the brain directly, thereby destroying the body's ability to function.

CRABS (PUBIC LICE) AND GENITAL WARTS

Pubic lice, also known as "crabs," are specific to humans and are passed from one person to another by sexual contact. They may be caught, too, by close contact with the infested bedding, towels, or clothing of an infected person.

They produce an intense itching of the skin beneath the pubic hair, sometimes only at night, and are easily spotted by close examination of the area, which reveals the tiny adult louse (pediculosis pubis) living between the hair roots, or the minute white eggs cemented firmly to the roots of the hair so that they cannot be easily dislodged.

TREATMENT   Simply washing with soap and water, no matter how thoroughly you do it, will not kill the crabs or dislodge the eggs that will hatch out to give you a whole new generation of the blood-sucking pests. Instead, use one of the many special shampoos or lotions, available from pharmacies, which are effective for the treatment of head lice (nits). There will be detailed instructions on the pack of the anti-nit treatment, but this is the usual routine:

- Follow the instructions written on the bottle of special shampoo or lotion to the letter.

- Change into clean clothes after using the shampoo or lotion, and thoroughly wash all your other clothes, bedding, towels, and washcloths before you next use them.

- When the treatment is complete, remove dead eggs from the hair with a fine metal- or plastic-toothed comb.

- If the itching does not subside immediately, repeat the treatment and the hair combing seven days later.

- Make sure you tell all your sexual contacts, and anyone in regular close contact with you, to treat themselves as a precaution.

GENITAL WARTS

Genital warts, like those that appear on the hands and elsewhere, are believed to be caused by a virus, the human papilloma virus. They are usually (but not always) transmitted by sexual contact with someone who already has them, and they appear, after an incubation period of four to 20 weeks, on the penis, the lips of the vagina, and in or around the anus. They may disappear spontaneously, but often recur.

Genital warts have been linked with cases of cervical cancer. A woman who has genital warts, or who has a partner with them, should have frequent Pap tests.

TREATMENT   Genital warts are fairly simple to treat by the application of a caustic substance, or by freezing or electrical cauterization, but should not be ignored because the virus that causes them is suspected of involvement in the onset of cancer of the cervix.

- If you discover a wart or warts in your genital or anal regions, consult your doctor or a venereal disease clinic as soon as possible, and do not have sex with anyone until the treatment is complete.

- Do not use over-the-counter preparations because the skin of the penis and vaginal areas is very sensitive.

- Keep the affected area as clean and dry as possible with regular washing, using a mild soap and then gently patting dry.

SAFE SEX

The notion of "safe sex" was first promoted in the 1980s as a response to the spread of AIDS, but practicing safe sex will help to protect you against sexually transmitted diseases in general and not just against AIDS. Safe sex is largely a matter of common sense combined with an awareness of the risks involved in different kinds of sexual activity.

HIGH-RISK SEXUAL ACTIVITIES:

- Any sexual act that draws blood, whether intentionally or accidentally
- Anal intercourse without using a condom
- Vaginal intercourse without using a condom
- Insertion of fingers or hand into the anus
- Sharing penetrative sex aids

MEDIUM-RISK SEXUAL ACTIVITIES:

- Anal intercourse with a condom
- Vaginal intercourse with a condom
- Cunnilingus
- Fellatio, especially to climax
- Anal kissing or licking
- Sexual activities involving urination
- Wet (tongue-to-tongue) kissing

LOW-RISK SEXUAL ACTIVITIES:

- Mutual masturbation (except cunnilingus and fellatio)
- Rubbing genitals against partner's body
- Dry kissing

NO-RISK SEXUAL ACTIVITIES:

- Non-genital massage
- Self-masturbation

———— USING A CONDOM ————

One of the chief weapons in combating the spread of sexual disease is the more widespread use of the condom. Though it does not guarantee complete protection, it does reduce the risks substantially.

The condom must be in place before any vaginal or anal penetration or oral sex takes place, and the penis needs to be fully erect.

Squeeze the receptacle end free of air and unroll the condom fully over the penis. To prevent it from bursting, do not stretch it tightly.

During withdrawal, hold the base of the condom to prevent semen from spilling. Use a new condom for each act of intercourse.

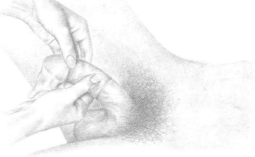

USEFUL ADDRESSES

USA

For general problems:

American Association
of Sex Educators, Counselors
and Therapists
Dupont Circle NW, Suite 220
Washington, D.C. 20036

Information Service
of the Kinsey Institute
for Sex Research
416 Morrison Hall
Indiana University
Bloomington, Ind. 47401

Institute for Family Research
and Education
760 Ostrom Avenue
Syracuse, N.Y. 13210

Sex Information and Education
Council of the U.S.
84 Fifth Ave.
New York, N.Y. 10011

National Women's Health Network
224 Seventh St. SE
Washington, D.C. 20003

**For disease prevention and
counseling:**

American Foundation for
the Prevention of
Venereal Disease, Inc.
335 Broadway
New York, N.Y. 10013

Centers for Disease Control
Bureau of State Services
Venereal Disease
Control Division
Atlanta, Ga. 30333

Gay Men's Health Crisis
129 W. 20 Street
New York, N.Y. 10011

Herpes Resource Center
P.O. Box 100
Palo Alto, Calif. 94302

For family planning :

Planned Parenthood
Federation of America
810 Seventh Ave.
New York, N.Y. 10019

National Clearinghouse for
Family Planning Information
P.O. Box 225
Rockville, Md. 20852

For sex throughout life:

American Association of
Retired Persons
1909 K Street NW
Washington, D.C. 20049

American Cancer Society
777 Third Ave.
New York, N.Y. 10017

American Heart Association
7320 Greenville Ave.
Dallas, Texas 75231

Arthritis Foundation
67 Irving Place
New York, N.Y. 10003

National Multiple
Sclerosis Foundation
205 E. 42 St.
New York, N.Y. 10017

Endometriosis Association
8585 North 76th Place
Milwaukee, Wis. 53223

This list is by no means
comprehensive but merely a
starting point for inquiries.
There are local organizations
dealing with family planning,
lesbian/gay issues, sexual
education, and counseling in
many communities.

CANADA

For general problems:

The Sex Information and
Education Council of Canada
(SIECCAN)
850 Coxwell Avenue
East York, Ontario M4C 5R1
Phone: (416) 466-5304

The Ontario Coalition
of Rape Crisis Centres
Box 1929
Peterborough, Ontario K9J 7X7
Phone: (705) 745-3646

For family planning:

Planned Parenthood
Federation of Canada
1 Nicholas Street, Suite 430
Ottawa, Ontario K1N 7B7
Phone: (613) 238-4474

Infertility Awareness Association
of Canada
104 -1785 Alta Vista Drive
Ottawa, Ontario K1G 3Y6
Phone: (613) 738-8968

**For PMS and other women's
health issues:**

Women's Health Centre
790 Bay Street, 8th Floor
Toronto, Ontario M5G 1N9
Phone: (416) 586-0211

For menopause:

A Friend Indeed:
For Women in the
Prime of Life
Box 515
Place du Parc Station
Montreal, Quebec H2W 2P1
Phone: (514) 843-5730

Canadian AIDS Society
30 Metcalfe Street, 6th Floor
Ottawa, Ontario K1N 7X2
Phone: (613) 230-3580

GLOSSARY

A

Abstinence In sexual terms, refraining from sexual intercourse.

Adolescence The period of human development that occurs between puberty and adulthood, when the individual is no longer a child but not yet an adult.

Adultery Sexual intercourse between a married man or woman and someone who is not his or her wife or husband; also called extramarital sex.

AIDS (Acquired Immune Deficiency Sydrome) A condition casued by the Human Immunodeficiency Virus (HIV) in which the body loses its ability to defend itself against illness.

Anal intercourse A form of sexual intercourse (either heterosexual or homosexual) in which a man inserts his penis into his partner's anus.

Androgens Hormones that promote the development of the male sexual organs and male secondary sexual characteristics. They are produced in large amounts in the testicles of men and in small amounts in the adrenal glands of both men and women, and regulate the level of sexual desire in both males and females. See also Testosterone.

Androgyne A person having both male and female characteristics, and incomplete male and female sexual organs. Also called a hermaphrodite.

Androgynous Having characteristics that are both masculine and feminine.

Anus The excretory opening at the end of the rectum.

Aphrodisiac Any substance, such as a food, drink, or drug, that is believed to stimulate or enhance sexual desire. The most effective ingredient of any alleged aphrodisiac is probably its reputation.

Areola The pigmented area around the human nipple, which swells slightly at times of sexual arousal.

Arousal Changes to the body, due to physical and mental stimuli, which prepare it for intercourse.

Asexual Having no apparent sex or sex organs.

B

Basal body temperature The normal termperature of the human body. A woman's basal body temperature rises just after ovulation, so by taking daily temperature readings a woman can detect when she has ovulated, and use this information in the termperature method of natural birth control.

Bestiality Sexual activity between a person and an animal; zoophilia.

Bigamy Illegally marrying a second wife or husband while still married to the first. See also Polyandry, Polygamy, Polygyny.

Birth control see Contraception.

Bisexual Being sexually attracted to people of both sexes and/or having sexual relations with them.

C

Calendar method A form of natural birth control in which the period of ovulation is calculated from the beginning of each menstrual period.

Candida A yeast infection of the vagina.

Carnal knowledge Sexual intercourse.

Castration Surgical removal of the male testicles or the female ovaries.

Celibacy An unmarried state or voluntary abstinence from sexual intercourse.

Cervical cancer Cancer of the cervix.

Cervical cap A contraceptive device which blocks the entrance to the cervix.

Cervical mucus method A form of natural birth control in which the period of ovulation is detected from changes in the nature of the mucus wihin the cervix.

Cervix The neck of the uterus; it connects the uterus with the vagina.

Chancre The visible symptom of primary syphilis.

Change of life The menopause.

Chastity Voluntary abstinence from all forms of sexual intercourse.

Chlamydia A sexually transmitted disease caused by a bacterium.

Circumcision A minor operation to remove the foreskin of the penis, usually performed for religious reasons or for reasons of hygiene, or to correct phimosis, a tight foreskin.

Climacteric The physical and psychological changes that accompany menopause in women.

Climax The point during sexual activity when orgasm is reached.

Clitoris The little, nose-shaped organ at the top of the small lips of a woman's vulva. It becomes erect when the woman is sexually stimulated, and because it contains many nerve endings, it is very sensitive to touch. It plays a large part in the process that leads to female orgasm.

Coitus Sexual intercourse.

Coitus interruptus Withdrawal of the penis from the vagina prior to ejaculation; a very risky method of contraception. Also called the withdrawal method.

Conception The fertilization of an ovum by a sperm.

Condom A thin rubber sheath placed over the erect penis before sexual intercourse to prevent sperm from entering the vagina; a female condom is a thin rubber tube, closed at one end, that is inserted into the vagina before intercourse to prevent sperm from entering the vagina.

Contraceptive Any device or medication, such as a condom or a hormonal pill, that is used to permit intercourse without conception.

Copulation Sexual intercourse.

Cowper's glands A pair of glands, near the prostate gland of a male, that produce a substance that neutralizes any acidity within the urethra (which could kill sperm) and becomes part of the seminal fluid; it also helps to lubricate the tip of the penis.

Crabs Pubic lice.

Cross-dressing Dressing in the clothing of the opposite sex. See also Transvestite.

Cunnilingus A form of oral sex in which the tongue or mouth is used to stimulate the vulva of a woman.

Cystitis Inflammation of the bladder caused by a bacterial infection.

D

Deviation Any form of sexual behavior considered to be abnormal.

Diaphragm A contraceptive device, made of thin rubber, placed over the cervix before sexual intercourse to prevent sperm from entering it.

Dildo An artificial erect penis used for female masturbation. See also Vibrator.

Douche A device for squirting a jet of water or other liquid into the vagina to cleanse it, or the liquid itself. Useless as a form of birth control and unnecessary for hygiene if the vagina is healthy.

Dysfunction In sexual terms, any problem — such as impotence or vaginismus — that interferes with sexual activity.

Dysmenorrhea Unusually difficult or painful menstruation, often involving cramps, nausea, headache, and other discomfort.

Dyspareunia Pain experienced by a woman during sexual intercourse, for instance because of involuntary tightening of the vaginal muscles.

E

Ejaculation The ejection of semen from the penis.

Endocrine glands The glands that produce hormones and secrete them into the bloodstream. They include the testicles and the ovaries.

Endometrium The lining of the uterus. If an egg is fertilized, it implants itself into the endometrium and begins to develop. Once a month, if no egg is implanted in it, the endometrium is discarded during the process of menstruation.

Epididymis One of the sets of tubes into which newly produced sperm pass from the testicle for storage and maturation, before entering the vas deferens ready for ejaculation.

Erection The swelling and stiffening of the penis, clitoris, or nipples during sexual stimulation.

Erogenous zones Those parts of the body, such as the breasts and genitals, that are especially sensitive to sexual stimulation.

Erotic Concerning or arousing sexual desire or pleasure. See also Pornography.

Estrogen Any of several steroid hormones secreted chiefly by a woman's ovaries. Estrogen stimulates the changes in a woman's reproductive organs during her monthly cycle, and promotes the development of the female secondary sex characteristics. Synthetic estrogen is used in some contraceptive pills; it causes ovulation to be suppressed.

Eunuch A man whose testicles have been removed.

Exhibitionist In sexual terms, a man who gets sexual pleasure from exposing his penis in public.

Extramarital sex Adultery.

F

Fallopian tubes The tubes that connect the ovaries with the uterus, and in which fertilization of ova occurs at conception.

Family planning The use of contraception to limit the size of a family.

Fantasy In sexual terms, imagining sexual situations or events involving real or imaginary people.

Fellatio A form of oral sex in which the tongue or mouth is used to stimulate the penis.

Fertile Capable of conception.

Fertile period The days during a woman's menstrual cycle when conception is possible.

Fertilization The penetration of the outer wall of an ovum by a sperm. Once fertilized, the ovum can begin its long development into a baby.

Fetishism A form of sexual behavior in which the handling of an inanimate object or of a part of the body other than the genitals is necessary for sexual satisfaction. Common fetish objects include rubber clothing, shoes, and feet.

Foreplay Sexual activity, including kissing and fondling, that provides stimulation prior to actual intercourse. See also Petting.

Foreskin The retractable fold of skin covering the tip of the penis; the prepuce.

Fornication Sexual intercourse between unmarried people.

French kissing Tongue-to-tongue kissing.

Frigidity A now discredited term for an inability to enjoy sexual intercourse.

G

Gay Homosexual.

Genital herpes A sexually transmitted disease caused by the herpes simplex virus.

Genitals The external sex organs: a man's penis and testicles; a woman's labia, clitoris, and vagina.

Genital warts see Venereal warts.

Glans The rounded, cone-shaped head of the penis.

Gonads See Sex glands.

Gonorrhea A sexually transmitted disease caused by a bacterium.

Group sex A number of people indulging in various sexual activities with each other at the same time. See also Orgy.

G spot The Grafenberg spot, a small area within the vagina that is especially responsive to stimulation.

H

Hermaphrodite see Androgyne.

Herpes see Genital Herpes.

Heterosexual Sexually attracted to people of the opposite sex.

HIV Human Immunodeficiency Virus, the virus that causes AIDS.

Homosexual Sexually attracted to people of the same sex as oneself.

Hormone A chemical substance produced by an endocrine gland. Some of these hormones — the sex hormones — play an important part in human sexual and reproductive functions. The sex hormones include androgen, estrogen, progesterone, and testosterone.

Hormone Replacement Therapy (HRT) The use of synthetic or natural hormones to counteract some of the effects of menopause.

Hot flashes An unpleasant symptom of menopause, consisting of sudden feelings of heat accompanied by heavy perspiration. Caused by changes in the blood vessels of the skin as a result of a drop in estrogen production.

Hymen A thin membrane that partly covers the entrance to the vagina in most females who have not had sexual intercourse.

I

Implantation The embedding of a fertilized ovum into the endometrium of the uterus.

Impotence A male sexual dysfunction involving the inability to achieve an erection or to maintain it for long enough to have intercourse or ejaculate.

Incest Sexual relations (heterosexual or homosexual) between close relatives, for example between father and daughter or brother and sister.

Infertility The inability of a woman to become pregnant, or of a man to impregnate a woman: sterility.

IUD (intrauterine device) A contraceptive device fitted within the uterus to prevent the implantation of a fertilized ovum into the endometrium.

L

Labia The lips of the female genitals. The small inner lips are called the labia minora, and the large outer lips the labia majora.

Lesbian A female homosexual.

Libido Sexual urge or desire.

M

Maidenhead An old name for the hymen.

Masochism A form of sexual behavior in which a person derives sexual pleasure from having pain inflicted on him or her. See also Sadism, Sadomasochism.

Masturbation Stimulation of one's own sexual organs, usually to achieve orgasm. Mutual masturbation is when partners stimulate each other's sexual organs, either to achieve orgasm or as a prelude to sexual intercourse.

Menarche The first occurrence of menstruation in a woman's life.

Menopause The period in a woman's life when menstruation ceases.

Menstruation The monthly discharge of the endometrium that takes place if no fertilized ovum has implanted in it.

Monilial vaginitis A yeast infection of the vagina.

'Morning after' pill A contraceptive pill, containing a very high dose of estrogen, that can prevent a pregnancy if taken within 72 hours of intercourse.

N

Natural birth control Avoiding pregnancy by abstaining from sexual intercourse on the days during the menstrual cycle when conception is possible, or by withdrawal of the penis from the vagina before ejaculation. Also called the "rhythm method" of birth control, a collective term that covers the calendar, cervical mucus and temperature methods that are used to determine which days are safe for sexual intercourse. See also Calendar method, Cervical mucus method, Coitus interruptus, Temperature method.

Nipple The tip of the breast; an important erogenous zone, it becomes erect during sexual arousal.

Noctural emission The involuntary ejaculation of semen during sleep; a wet dream.

NSU (Nonspecific urethritis) A common sexually transmitted disease caused by bacteria.

O

Onanism An old name for masturbation.

Oral contraceptive The Pill.

Oral sex Using the mouth to stimulate the genitals of a partner. Also called oral-genital sex, it includes both cunnilingus and fellatio.

Orgasm The most intense part (climax) of sexual excitement, involving extremely pleasurable sensations and usually, in the male, ejaculation.

Orgy A wild, abandoned gathering usually involving group sex, excessive drinking, and sometimes consumption of illicit substances. See also Group sex.

Ova Eggs; the word "ovum" refers to a single egg, and "ova" is the plural and refers to two or more eggs. Both words are of Latin origin.

Ovary One of the two female sex glands that produce ova (eggs) and the sex hormones estrogen and progesterone.

Ovulation The monthly release of an ovum from an ovary. The ovum passes into one of the Fallopian tubes where it awaits fertilization by a sperm.

Ovum An egg; two or more are referred to as ova.

P

Pedophilia Sexual activities between adults and children of either sex.

Pap test A test which is used for detecting diseases of the vagina or uterus, especially cancer of the cervix. A sample of mucus is taken from, for example, the opening of the cervix, and smeared onto a glass slide so that it can be examined under a microscope. The Pap test is named after its inventor, George Papanicolaou.

Pederasty Homosexual activities of men and boys.

Pelvic inflammatory disease (PID) A potentially serious disease affecting women and usually the result of untreated sexually transmitted diseases such as gonorrhea or chlamydia.

Penile Of or relating to the penis.

Penis The erectile male sex organ.

Perineum In women, the area between the vagina and the anus; in men, the area between the scrotum and the anus.

Period Menstruation.

Perversion Any unusual means of obtaining sexual gratification.

Petting Sexual activity, such as caressing the breasts or genitals, either instead of, or as a prelude, to sexual intercourse.

Phallic Of or relating to the penis, usually when it is in the erect state.

Phallus Another name for a penis, usually referring to an erect one.

Pheromones Substances secreted by the body that have an odor, not always noticeable, that stimulate sexual desire in members of the opposite sex.

Phimosis An abnormal tightness of the foreskin that prevents it from being pulled back over the head of the penis. It often can be corrected by gentle stretching, but circumcision may be needed.

Pill The type of contraceptive medication taken by mouth, containing synthetic hormones that prevent pregnancy.

Pituitary gland The body's master endocrine gland. Situated at the base of the brain, it secretes hormones that regulate the action of the testicles and the ovaries, other endocrine glands.

Platonic relationship A close relationship between two people that does not involve sexual activity.

Polyandry Marriage between one woman and two or more men at the same time.

Polygamy Having more than one wife or husband at a time.

Polygyny Marriage between one man and two or more women at the same time.

Pornography Written or other material designed to stimulate sexual excitement. In general, "hard-core" pornography explicitly describes or depicts sexual acts such as intercourse, whereas "soft-core" pornography usually describes or depicts men or women in sexually provocative poses or situations. See also Erotic.

Premarital sex Sexual intercourse between two people who intend to marry, or simply between two unmarried people. See also Adultery.

Premature ejaculation A sexual dysfunction in which a man ejaculates before, or immediately after, inserting his penis into his partner's vagina.

Progesterone The female sex hormone that prepares the uterus to receive and sustain a fertilized ovum.

Progestin The synthetic equivalent of progesterone

used in contraceptives.

Promiscuity Having a number of different sexual partners, usually on a casual basis.

Prostate gland A gland that surrounds the urethra of a man. It seals off the exit from the bladder to prevent urine escaping while the penis is erect, and produces one of the main constituents of semen. Contractions of its muscles and others around it pump the semen through the urethra and out of the penis during ejaculation.

Prostitute Someone who provides sexual services in exchange for money.

Puberty The beginning of adolescence, during which a boy begins to ejaculate semen and a girl begins to menstruate.

Pubic hair The hair around the genitals.

Pubic lice Lice that live in the pubic hair. They are usually caught by sexual contact with an infected person; also called crabs.

R

Rape To force someone to have sexual intercourse against their will.

Rectum The lower end of the large intestine, which ends at the anus.

Refractory period The period after orgasm during which, for most men and some women, further sexual response is temporarily inhibited.

Reproductive system Those parts of the human body that are directly involved in reproduction.

Rhythm method see Natural birth control.

Rubber A condom.

S

Sadism A form of sexual behavior in which a person derives sexual pleasure from inflicting pain on another person. See also Sadomasochism, Masochism.

Sadomasochism A form of sexual behavior in which a person derives sexual pleasure from a combination of sadism and masochism. See also Sadism, Masochism.

Safe period The days during a woman's monthly cycle when sexual intercourse is least likely to result in pregnancy. See also Natural birth control.

Safe sex Forms of sexual activity that carry a relatively low risk of contracting sexually transmitted diseases (especially AIDS).

Scrotum The pouch of loose, wrinkled skin that contains a man's testicles.

Secondary sexual characteristics The physical characteristics, apart from the main reproductive organs, that develop during puberty and differentiate men from women.

Seduction To persuade someone to engage in sexual intercourse.

Semen The mixture of sperm and seminal fluid ejaculated from a man's penis during orgasm.

Seminal fluid One of the main constituents of semen; produced mainly by the prostate gland.

Seminal vesicle Either of two small pouches at the back of a man's prostate gland that discharge seminal fluid into the urethra.

Sex-change operation A surgical operation available to a transsexual man or woman that enables him or her to become, as nearly as possible, a member of the opposite sex.

Sex glands The ovaries of a woman or the testicles of a man. Also called gonads.

Sex hormones Hormones secreted by the sex glands which affect the characteristics and behavior of males and females. The principal sex hormones are androgen and estrogen.

Sex organs The internal and external organs that differentiate men from women, including the genitals and the sex glands.

Sexual intercourse Sexual activity in which the man inserts his erect penis into the vagina of his partner. See also Anal intercourse.

Sexually transmitted disease A disease that is passed from one person to another by sexual activity. Sexually transmitted diseases (STDs) include gonorrhea, syphilis, AIDS, and chlamydia. The term "sexually transmitted disease" has largely replaced the older term "venereal disease" (VD).

Sixty-nine A slang term for two people simultaneously engaging in oral sex with each other; the positions they adopt when doing this resemble the number 69, when viewed from the side.

Smegma A smelly, cheeselike substance that accumulates under the foreskin of an uncircumcised man (or under the hood of a woman's clitoris) because of poor hygiene.

Sodomy Anal intercourse.

Sperm The male reproductive cell. Its purpose is to fertilize the ovum of a woman and thus initiate pregnancy. Millions of sperm are produced in the testicles and mixed with seminal fluid for ejaculation from the penis.

Spermicide Any specially formulated substance that is placed in the vagina before intercourse, or used in conjuction with a condom or diaphragm, to kill sperm and so act as a contraceptive.

Squeeze technique A method of curing premature ejaculation in which a man's partner squeezes the head of his penis just before he reaches the point at which ejaculation is inevitable.

STD Abbreviation for Sexually Transmitted Disease.

Sterilization Any event that makes a person unable to bear or produce a child. Sterilization may be deliberate, for example by means of an operation such as tubal ligation or a vasectomy, or it may occur as a complication of a sexually transmitted disease if treatment is neglected or delayed.

Stop-start technique A method by which a man can teach himself to avoid premature ejaculation, by temporarily stopping all stimulation when he feels that he is reaching the point at which ejaculation is inevitable. See also Squeeze technique.

Straight An informal term meaning heterosexual, as opposed to homosexual.

Syphilis A sexually transmitted disease caused by a bacterium.

T

Temperature method A form of natural birth control in which the period of ovulation is detected from changes in the body temperature.

Testicles The two male sex glands, carried in the scrotum, that manufacture sperm and produce sex hormones. Also called testes (singular: testis).

Testosterone The primary male sex hormone (or androgen) produced by the testicles. It is responsible for the male sex drive and the male secondary sexual characteristics. Testosterone is also produced by the adrenal glands of both men and women, and in women it is responsible for the female sex drive. See also Androgens.

Transsexual A man or woman who feels that he or she is really a member of the opposite sex, trapped in the wrong body. Transsexuals may undergo sex change operations and hormone treatment to change the sex of their bodies.

Transvestite A man (or, sometimes, a woman) who has a strong compulsion to cross-dress (to dress in the clothing of the opposite sex). For many transvestites, cross-dressing is necessary for them to be able to enjoy sexual activity.

Trichomoniasis An infection of the vagina, often sexually transmitted.

Tubal ligation A method of female sterilization in which the Fallopian tubes are cut so that ova cannot pass down them or sperm pass up.

U

Urethra The tube through which urine is passed from the bladder. In men, the urethra is also the channel through which semen is ejaculated.

Urethritis Inflammation of the urethra, caused by an infection. See also NSU.

Uterus The womb; the organ of a woman in which the fertilized ovum is deposited and where it develops into a baby. See also Endometrium.

V

Vagina The soft, short passage that leads from a woman's vulva to her cervix, and into which the penis is inserted during sexual intercourse.

Vaginitis An inflammation of the vagina.

Vaginismus A condition in which the muscles around the vagina contract tightly, making sexual intercourse difficult or impossible.

Vas deferens Either of the two tubes (vasa deferentia) that convey sperm from the testicles.

Vasectomy A method of male sterilization in which the vasa deferentia are cut so that sperm cannot pass along them and into the semen.

VD Abbreviation for Venereal Disease.

Venereal disease Old term for sexually transmitted disease.

Venereal warts Small warts on or around the genitals; may be sexually transmitted.

Vibrator A battery-operated device, usually penis-shaped, that vibrates and is used to stimulate the clitoris or the vagina, either for masturbation or as a prelude to sexual intercourse. See also Dildo.

Virgin Any person, male or female, who has not had sexual intercourse.

Voyeurism A form of sexual behavior in which a person gets sexual pleasure from watching the sexual activities of other people, or even from watching other people getting undressed.

Vulva The external sex organs of a woman.

W Y Z

Water sports Sexual activities involving urination.

Wet dream The involuntary ejaculation of semen during sleep; nocturnal emission.

Withdrawal method see Coitus interruptus.

Womb The uterus.

Yeast infection An infection of the vagina, such as candida, caused by a yeastlike fungus.

Zoophilia A rare form of sexual behavior involving sexual contact with animals; bestiality.

INDEX

ACKNOWLEDGMENTS

Editorial Director: Amy Carroll
Creative Director: Denise Brown
Art Editor: Tracy Timson
Designers: Earl Neish, Phillip Tarver
U.S. Editor: Laaren Brown Hort

Editorial Assistance: Elizabeth Thompson
Madeline Weston
Ian Wood

Computer Output: Rowena Feeny
Howard Pemberton & Lincolnshire College of
    Art and Design
Frances Prà-Lopez
Deborah Rhodes

Production Controller: Antony Heller

Photographs: Paul Robinson, David Murray

Illustrations: Sue Linney (*pages 14-15, 78-79, 80, 82, 152, 165, 167, 208, 211, 225, 245*)

Howard Pemberton (*pages 18-19, 22-23, 26-27, 218-219*)

Kuo Kang Chen (*pages 34-35, 98-99, 100-101, 102-103, 194-195, 202-203, 204-205, 206-207*)

Special Thanks to: Thad Yablonsky, M.D.